# Ikkuma: Evolution *of* Vitality

GARY LeBLANC

BURMAN BOOKS
MEDIA CORP.

Copyright © 2013 Ikkuma: Evolution of Vitality

Published by BurmanBooks Media Corp.
260 Queens Quay West
Suite 904
Toronto, Ontario
Canada M5J 2N3

All rights reserved. No part of this publication may be reproduced, stored in a retrieval system, or transmitted in any form by any process—electronic, photocopying, recording, or otherwise—without the prior written consent of BurmanBooks Media Corp.

*Cover:* Tommy Carlson
*Editing:* Anna Watson
*Illustrations:* Sheila LeBlanc

*Distribution:*
TruMedia Group LLC
575 Prospect Street, Suite 301
Lakewood, NJ 08701

ISBN 978-1-927005-36-1

The book may contain health-related and medical-related information including statements of facts, views, opinions, recommendations, descriptions of, or references to, products, services and treatments. Such health-related and medical-related information made available by BurmanBooks Media Corp. and the books authors and contributors is: (a) for informational purposes only; (b) not to be used or construed as a substitute for medical or any other professional advice, diagnosis, or treatment; and (c) not intended as a recommendation or endorsement of any specific tests, products, procedures, opinions or any other information. Reliance on any health-related or medical-related information in the book is solely at your own risk. Always seek the advice of your physician or other qualified health provider with any questions you may have regarding a medical or health condition. Never disregard professional medical advice or delay in seeking it because of something you have read in this book. You agree that all risk associated with the use of, or reliance on, any of the information in this book rests with you. You further agree that neither the author nor the contributor nor BurmanBooks Media Corp. shall be responsible or liable, directly or indirectly, in any way for any loss or damage of any kind incurred as a result of, or in connection with, your use of, or reliance on, any such information.

*Dedicated to Brad MacMillan*

## Acknowledgments

Writing this was definitely a journey out of my comfort zone. I'd like to thank the people critical in making it happen:

My business partner Brian Coones. What can I say... There wouldn't be a book without Brian's vision. My brother always.

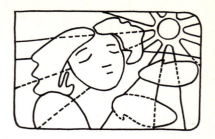

**"Gratitude"**—The key to being grateful is reviewing what you have. I am grateful for the incredible people who have helped me on this amazing transformation.

Angelina and I bounced concepts around until they were sound. I couldn't think of anybody better to collaborate with.

Kennedy Lodato for being the fitness guru!

Sarah Moritz got me through countless moments of doubt and was the editor behind the scenes.

My sisters! Jacqueline for her engagement on the project from day one and Sheila for the amazing illustrations that truly pay homage to Inuit culture.

Don for taking the time to be a fantastic sounding board and ambassador!

The rest of my family and friends. When everyone believes in you more than you believe in yourself, you don't want to let them down.

THANK YOU!

# Table of Contents

Acknowledgments  v
Foreword  1
Prologue  5
Introduction  15

## Section ONE

### Part One—How the Body Works  20

Our Body's Fuel  20
Food Building Blocks—Macronutrients  24
Hormones… The Body's Chemical Messengers  38
Now It's Feeding Time!  40
Digestion  42
I Have a 'Gut' Feeling  49

### Part Two—Disease… Know Thy Enemy  57

Key Precursors to Disease  58
Common Diseases  71
Cancer  75
Diabetes  82
Cardiovascular Disease and Stroke  87

## Section TWO
**Part One: Foods To 'Live' By**
*(Ikkuma Translation: Feeding the Fire)* **90**

Key Foods to Eat 95
To Be or Not to Be Organic 120
So What About Supplements? 148
Eat Your Power Foods 168
Alkaline Versus Acidic Foods... WTF? **171**

**Part Two: Foods To 'Drive' By**
*(Ikkuma Translation: The Fire Is Starting to Fade)* **180**

## Section THREE
**Toxins... The Ugly Truth**
*(Ikkuma Translation: 'Get That Tire Out of the Fire!')* **208**

The Marvels of Modern Medicine? 236

## Section FOUR
**Keeping the Body Tuned Up**
*(Ikkuma Translation: Stoking the Fire)* **254**

Stress... The Silent Killer 256
Sleep... The Body's Time to Heal 264
Fitness... Use It or Lose It 274
In the End It's Your Choice... 306

Bibliography 311

# Foreword

I got to know Gary several years ago during a time when one of his best friends was diagnosed with cancer. Being an engineer, Gary tried to grasp the issues surrounding cancer and understand the latest thoughts concerning prevention and treatment. Eventually Gary became interested in identifying how the body works and how it is impacted by external factors such as the environment, nutrition, exercise, and so on.

When I first heard that Gary was going to write a book about health I was extremely pleased and excited to see the final copy. I had already sat through two seminars by Gary where he covered his thoughts on exercise, nutrition, and supplements. Not only was the information interesting and valuable but Gary's understanding of the research when answering questions during the seminars was extremely impressive. I have personally taken his advice on exercise, supplements and diet and have been pleased with the results.

What I really appreciate about the book is the amount of work that Gary has put into understanding the latest thinking on how our body functions, how it processes nutrients and what each of us can do to avoid illness.

My personal philosophy is that we need to have balance in our lives whether that be work, fitness, developing our mind or having fun. It all eventually boils down to where we choose to spend our time and how do we do things in the most efficient way possible to obtain the results we desire. Each of us are individuals on this journey of life. We need to take control of what we do with our time, how we treat others, and also importantly, how we treat ourselves.

As Gary points out, if someone does not take an interest in their own wellbeing they cannot expect someone else, their family or the government to do it for them. They will live with the consequences. We only have one body and one brain, so why not take reasonable actions to ensure that we have a functional mind and body and a positive attitude.

I find the amount of information that is available about diet, supplements, exercise, the impact of toxins and what we put on our body, sleep, and so on is not only confusing but extremely time consuming to sift through. What I love about Gary's book is that he has taken an unbiased view and spent countless hours researching a wide variety of topics which he has summarized in a very readable fashion so that we can all have a good understanding of how things work and what we can be doing to optimize our health.

For anyone to do this on their own it would take hundreds if not thousands of hours to review the latest research to sift through what makes sense, what is fact-based and what is opinion, and analytically come to a conclusion about what is best for ourselves. Gary has done this for us. I have no doubt there are other opinions in specific fields and our knowledge in this area will continue to evolve and grow. However, I am confident that the conclusions Gary has reached are based on his unbiased, detailed research.

To the readers of this book, if you ever have the pleasure of meeting Gary and listening to one of his presentations, he is not only passionate but also very generous with his time in talking to people and answering questions to make them more educated in these fields. Moreover, he is a living example of how to be in great shape and practices what he preaches.

One of the most important part of anyone's life is to be positive. We have so much to live for, so why not invest the time to understand how to maximize the functioning of our body and mind? This leads to a healthy spirit. It is relatively easy to live proactively in a way that keeps us optimally functioning in both body and spirit. It is amazing the number of people who show great discipline and attention to detail when they are at work—why not do the exact same for our most important asset—ourselves? I look forward to seeing if Gary can produce some natural products that lives up to the standards written about in the book such that we can eat and drink what is healthy and has been well researched.

I hope that you enjoy the book as much as I did. Additionally, I hope you gain the knowledge and motivation to apply whatever makes sense for you and that you live a happier, healthier life with less risk of developing a disease.

Gary, thank you for putting this book together. I know I was one of the people encouraging you to do so, so that we all could learn from it.

Don Walker
Chief Executive Officer
Magna International Inc.

*"Time is the coin of your life. It is the only coin you have, and only you can determine how it will be spent. Be careful lest you let other people spend it for you."*
—CARL SANDBERG, AMERICAN POET

# Prologue

This is for you Brad.

About six years ago a dear friend of mine, Brad MacMillan was diagnosed with non-Hodgkins lymphoma. The tragic diagnosis shocked his family and friends as Brad was a healthy, 42 year old man who ran every day and took care of his body. I watched him fight for three years until he succumbed to the disease on Mother's Day in 2010. Watching him struggle through the side effects was very difficult, however it was the chemotherapy itself that had the deepest impact on me. The pain and suffering he endured was beyond tolerable. No human being should ever go through something so unnatural and violent. Brad was administered so many needles that a central line to the heart was required. It became apparent to me that disease is not a natural state of being, but a tragic circumstance created by our modern environment.

It was at that moment that the little guy in my head snapped and asked what the hell was going on. When did our future become a sick game of Russian roulette? The difference with this game is, well, try loading the gun with five bullets instead of one. That's the future we're looking at if shit doesn't change.

Needless to say, Brad had a profound effect on me, but I was ashamed that it took his death for me to wake up and reassess how I was treating my body and living my life. Sure, up until that point I was in good shape but that was simply because I was vain. This vanity was stoked by years of stuttering as a kid and being called "dumbo" because my ears stuck out, which definitely took a toll on my self-confidence. I have since lost the stutter, got my ears pinned back and have done everything in my power to not only never be ridiculed again, but to do everything imaginable to be the best at everything I do. As you can imagine, this all came with a huge chip on my shoulder.

Unfortunately it took Brad's passing for me to lose that chip on my shoulder and embrace a more sustainable path to long lasting health. Someone shouldn't need to die for change to happen. Don't wait for your Brad! Get your head out of your ass and decide to take control.

Let's fast-forward a few years after Brad to the genesis of this book, and our company, *Ikkuma*. Ikkuma means fire in Inuit—an indigenous Canadian language. There are many reasons for this name, both in the language and its meaning. The Inuit are a very spiritual culture that feel a connection to all living things, and believe strongly in the power of words. There is therefore no better language to pay tribute to fire such a powerful and critical force of nature.

I find it unfortunate that fire has become vilified as a destructive force when, traditionally speaking, it has been linked to rejuvenation and rebirth. Fire is what occurs when the earth releases energy it has collected from the sun over many years. Not only is it an inspiring example of the sun's force, it performs a critical role in the cycle of all living things. For instance, a dead and diseased forest can lay dormant for hundreds of years without any growth. Within days after a forest fire however, poking through the destruction, this same forest will already show signs of new life.

Ikkuma—pronounced *ee-koo-ma*—ravages thousands of square miles of forest every day. The connection humans have with nature can be exemplified by the parallels that exist between the forests and ourselves. Similar to a dying forest, modern society has found itself plagued by disease and illness; if left untreated, these destructive realities will continue to worsen. Just as a fire brings a forest back to life, *Ikkuma: Evolution of Vitality* seeks to awaken the public, igniting a movement out of disease, toward renewed, healthy growth. This isn't a fad diet or a get well quick scheme. This book represents your get-out-of-jail-free card. Applying the logical and sustainable Ikkuma principles is the best chance you have to truly rewrite your future.

While it may feel daunting, this is not a process that will take years—simple changes today can physiologically change your health within days. You will be creating a new life for yourself; one with sustained energy, where you wake up feeling refreshed rather than lazy and lethargic, and where your body will be capable of activities it could not perform before. You will be living with the positivity and drive you were previously lacking. These changes are available for anyone to embrace. This book is a simple guide, giving you the tools to get there—now!

You may now be asking, who the hell am I and why should you even listen to me? Good question. First off, I have two degrees from a great school. They have given me the tools to effectively research and formulate concise call-to-actions. I'm also a life-coach and certified personal trainer. Specifically for Ikkuma, I have spent several years reading, researching, interviewing, and speaking about the body, the effects food has on the body, and how lack of exercise can destroy a body. I have sifted through books, articles, and lectures, and have undergone years of trial and error to extract what I truly consider to be the most important lessons and advice for physically, and psychologically, healthy living. So, yeah, I might not be a doctor, but ask yourself, does it take a doctor to analyze data and make logical recommendations? No.

Even though I just harped about not needing a doctor to write this book, I do have a fantastic doctor collaborating with me on Ikkuma—Angelina Riopel. She's a naturopathic doctor and has been my holistic sounding board throughout. In reality she is the good cop to my bad. In that, at times I may rant out of passion—respectfully—but I can always count on Angelina to reel me in. You'll notice when this happens. The ranting is definitely all me. I apologize in advance if my language may come off as offensive. This is not my goal. Let's just say that instead of an angry face emoticon, I'll just say what's on my mind. This will not be gratuitous swearing just for the sake of it. I truly do believe a "shit" here and there will give the requisite level of emphasis. In any event, I was born in Cape Breton, Nova Scotia, and "shit" seemed to be in my daily vernacular.

This book is broken down into 4 main sections:

- The body, basic physiology and disease—how it all works

- What you put in your body—good and bad food habits, including ingested toxins
- What you put on your body—topical toxins and other environmental factors
- How you treat your body—sleep, stress and fitness

Since I want this book to be a reference, these concepts are broken down into dozens of digestible sections, allowing you to pick up the book without feeling required to invest significant amounts of time to gain a benefit.

Woven into various sections of the book you will find **Ikkuma Info** sections—little pearls of information that relate to the material being presented. They are typically meant to stand alone and offer further perspective.

My overall goal was to create a book for everyday people—people who are busy and not yet able, or perhaps even willing, to invest extensive time learning how to improve their health and wellness. This book is not meant to be entirely prescriptive, but is simply an attempt to provide people with the tools they need to make decisions that are right for them—basically to wake everyone up! Change is the only option. The time is now to make a change. A new reality begins today.

Before I get too far down the rabbit hole let's put our society in context. There are four types of people who may hear about this book, namely, those who don't give a shit and may or may not be informed, and you guessed it, those who do give a shit and may or may not be informed. I call it the "Give A Shit" grid:

**"Give A Shit" Grid**

| Don't GAS (Give A Shit)/informed | GAS/informed |
|---|---|
| Don't GAS/not informed | GAS/not informed |

This book will leave the people who don't give a shit and are informed in the lurch (the top left hand quadrant). I choose to focus my time on the other three quadrants. First off, my goal is to make the book compelling enough that those who aren't informed—at both ends of the give a shit scale—will want to become informed. For those who give a shit and are informed, well, I know you will still learn a ton from reading *Ikkuma*. That makes my sample size pretty darn big, so unless you have a death wish or want to live with disease, this book will shock you into making changes. Ipso facto, this book has the potential to transform a generation.

We all need to answer the most important question: "How do I want to live?" Note that I didn't say "how *long*" do I want to live, but simply *"how"* do I want to live? It is important to be honest with yourself and reflect on why you have chosen to take this journey toward a healthy lifestyle. Whether it's to look better, to improve heart health, or to simply age with energy and vitality, this book will help you get there.

As I will repeat throughout this book, it is important to recognize that, because studies are imperfect by nature, most of the information that is presented to us will represent the best of our understanding today. The purpose of *Ikkuma: Evolution Of Vitality* then, is to sift through all the information we are smothered with and propose logical solutions.

This is not rocket science. Look at it as a health bank account. Let's call it your Ikkuma Account. I would venture a guess and say that most of you reading this have made a lot more health withdrawals than deposits. Maybe you're not the focus of a reality show for spending gone wrong, but you may definitely be in an overdraft situation. So, when you whine to me about not being able to eat cookies, first question the state of your Ikkuma Account and ask yourself if you can afford the withdrawal. When you get to where you need to be—your Ikkuma Account is balanced—you'll be in a position to have more flexibility regarding where you choose to make deposits and withdrawals. Until you get there, however, you're going to have to suck it up and sacrifice. That includes those idiotic "cheat" days. What the hell is a cheat day anyway? How can you cheat your way to a balanced account? It just doesn't makes sense. Like I said, get your Ikkuma Account in order first.

Here's a little set of equations for the visual readers:

### EXAMPLE #1: Overdrawn Ikkuma Account (a.k.a. "The Shitshow")

| | |
|---|---|
| Withdrawals: | (15 years of eating trash) |
| Deposits: | A multivitamin |
| Balance: | (your health is a mess) |
| Solution: | Stop stuffing your face with empty processed junk and clean up your act the Ikkuma way. In 12 weeks your account should be in much better standing |

### EXAMPLE #2: Healthy Ikkuma Account (a.k.a. "Abundant Vitality")

| | |
|---|---|
| Withdrawals: | (The odd late night munchies) |
| Deposits: | Wholesome organic nutrition and regular exercise |
| Balance: | Healthy enough to absorb the odd indulgence |
| Solution: | Pay attention to your body as you age and adjust accordingly. A mirror and how you physically, and mentally, feel are all you |

> need to let you know if you start making
> too many withdrawals.

Look, you can either apply the principles in the book or continue making withdrawals. It's not my place to bitch at you or hold your hand. If you aren't already gravely concerned about the future then maybe you need to have a reality check. This book may be the reality check that changes your life.

In the end, it boils down to common sense but I will still give you a ton of tools to get where you need to be; tools that will get you to that steady state where you can start making informed decisions about your health.

Beyond this book, what my partner Brian and I strive to achieve with Ikkuma Inc. (www.ikkuma.com) is to expand on Ikkuma's offerings. Through all of our interests—from this book to our health related products—we aim to improve the quality of as many lives as we can. Ikkuma will be synonymous with trust, authenticity, and integrity.

Success for me would be to inspire you to want to learn more, continually strive to be aware of your choices, and focus on living a happy and healthy life. I hope you enjoy it...

# Introduction

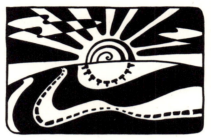

**"Beginnings"—The journey you are about to embark on is unique, but every journey does have a Beginning. Let's begin…**

*"It is no measure of health to be well adjusted to a profoundly sick society."*
—JIDDU KRISHNAMURTI, 20TH CENTURY INDIAN PHILOSOPHER

Throughout the book I will often refer to the "Western" diet epidemic. I am referring to both Americans and Canadians alike. I'll also quote facts that may refer to one country or the other. For all intents and purposes, both our countries are facing the same challenges in varying degrees. In order to put the present situation in context, let's look at a some shocking stats.

While America spends more per capita on health care than any other country in the world (nearly double that of Germany, who is next in line),

- over two thirds of the population is overweight (body mass index over 25),
- over one third is obese (body mass index over 30),
- over 25 million of its citizens have diabetes, and
- over 75 million are pre-diabetic (American Diabetes Association).

Note that some of these facts refer to body mass index or BMI. BMI is simply a measurement used to classify levels of obesity. Over 25 BMI is classified as overweight, which would describe someone at 5'9" weighing approximately 170 lbs and over 30 BMI is classified as obese, describing someone at the same height but weighing approximately 192 lbs.

At present rates of obesity, by 2030 nearly half of America's citizens will be obese. Maybe more alarming is that nearly a third of America's children are considered overweight and over 15% are obese—and this isn't just America's problem. Accordingly to Dr. Ezzati, Imperial College professor in London, in 2008 one third of the global population was overweight (potentially obese)—double the rates observed in 1980. (*Economist*—December 15, 2012).

This is both disappointing and disgusting at the same time. This isn't about vanity and being skinny, it's about a lost generation. A generation lost to disease! When are we going to wake the hell up?

Other statistics are equally as alarming:

- The American Cancer society reports that over 1 in 2 American males will get cancer in their lifetime; with females faring slightly better at over 1 in 3. (*Cancer Statistics* 2013, American Cancer Society, 2013)
- Diabetes (mostly type II) has been skyrocketing—strongly correlated with the obesity epidemic. As mentioned, over one out of every thirteen Americans now has some form of diabetes. Of those, nearly 30% are not even aware they have it. The health costs related to this epidemic in the U.S. is approximately $245 billion. (American Diabetes Association)

Pharmaceuticals are sold with the goal of improving these existing health problems, yet we are rarely informed that these conditions could have actually been avoided in the first place. So why is it that only the symptoms and not prevention are widely discussed? Well, pharmaceutical companies can't make money unless you are buying and relying on their drugs. To make matters worse, these drugs we so desperately rely on cause hundreds of adverse reactions; leading to the death of over 100,000 Americans annually. (Lazarou J, Pomeranz B, and Corey PN. "Incidence of adverse drug reactions in hospitalized patients." *JAMA 279* (1998): 1200–1205).

Not only do we over-medicate, but reliance on mechanically-made foods is also at an all-time high. Despite the genius behind nature's design of food, we have brushed it aside, allowing ourselves to be romanced by health claims hurled at us by food manufacturing companies.

Do you honestly think that any of the major processed food companies give a rat's ass that you won't be able to pay for your medical bills due to diabetes? They sure don't, but the one thing you can be sure off is that they'll market the hell out of their products—often directly to your children. Yeah, we should all be ashamed. When did society decide to value profits above the health of our children?

The simple truth is that the basis to healthy living lies in the recognition that nature has laid everything out for us. Throughout *Ikkuma: Evolution of Vitality* you will see one recurring theme—*we've had the solution to a vibrant and healthy life all this time, but have chosen to ignore it*. Sometimes the treasure lies right under our noses.

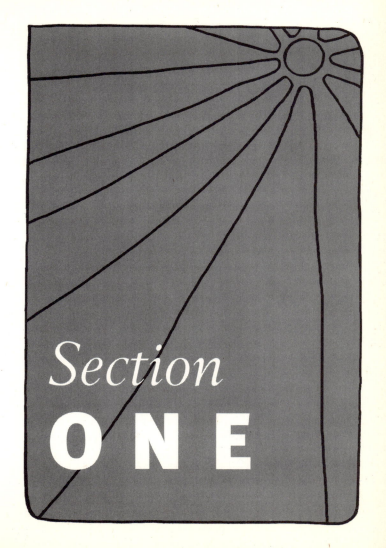

# *Part* **ONE**
## How the Body Works

*(Ikkuma Translation: Building The Fire)*

Hmmmmm, how the body works…do you even care? If you don't, then skip this section. Some people don't need to understand the 'why', they just want the 'what' and 'how'. That's perfectly fine. So, for those who don't care what happens in the body, I'll see you in the next section. But for those who want to truly be informed, bear with me through the theory in this section, because it will really drive home the necessity for change. Trust me, a little knowledge goes a long way. What you will read is logical. That's why you're going to love it so much. And like I said, I've done all the heavy lifting. You just need to kick back and start learning about how your amazingly intricate body works.

## Our Body's Fuel

### Brief history

The agricultural revolution, which occurred approximately 12,000 years ago, set the stage for a monumental shift in human evolution. In his book, *The Paleo Solution* (2010 Victoria Belt Publishing) Cordain discusses the effects this huge change in lifestyle had on our physical evolution and health.

Along with many others, Cordain contends that prior to this era, human beings were as tall as, and healthier than, present day humans. The rates of degenerative diseases were a fraction of what we see today, their skin was healthier, and they thrived physically. Furthermore, societies that have remained hunter-gatherers have consistently demonstrated better health than their farming counterparts, with lower mortality rates, fewer cavities, and longer life.

Now let's fast forward to the 21st century; after 12,000 years of progress, do we place value on what we feed our bodies? If what North Americans spend on food expenditures is any indication, we haven't. In 2010 Americans spent under 10% of their disposable income on eating: with approximately 5.5% of that going toward eating in the home, and 4% toward eating out (USDA Economic Research Service, Food CPI AND Expenditures). The percentage spent eating in the home is less than half of most countries, with Italy and France spending nearly three times more than Americans.

This is a massive digression from the 1930's, when nearly 25% of Americans' disposable income went to food. Obviously there have been advances in food technology, but this represents a small percentage of the decline. Western society, specifically North Americans, has chosen to produce and consume cheaper food of poor nutritional quality over buying high quality, non-genetically modified foods, void of contaminants. Ironically, although we may proportionately spend less on food in North America versus other parts of the world, we are one of the heaviest regions.

As reported in the HBO documentary series, *The Weight of a Nation*, the daily caloric consumption in the U.S. has risen in the past few decades from under 2200 calories to approximately 2700 calories. This startling rise of nearly 25% is entirely due to what we eat—cheap, high caloric food—and our sedentary lifestyles. There are no two ways about it, we have become a society that values iPods over our future health. You never hear people complain about the price of an iPod but people are appalled by the relatively high cost of organic food. Really? We spend a pittance on our food and then justify going on the cheap by convincing ourselves that a little pesticide is all right. What the heck, the corporations selling the pesticides say it's okay.

Not only is our "cheap" food essentially void of nutrition, but it hides the true cost. The subsidies—government financial support—on certain crops and environmental costs are not built into the price when you're paying less than a dollar for a two litre bottle of soda. Therein lies the irony: despite the fact it's making us sicker, processed and genetically modified food hoards the lion's share of all food subsidies. These subsidies mainly support commodities, crop insurance, conservation and disaster protection—and most of these crops are genetically modified. Out of the $277 billion in subsidies paid out between 1995–2011 in the U.S., corn, wheat, cotton and soy represented approximately $175 billion of the total payout. As will be shown later in the book, these crops are predominantly born of genetically modified seeds.

These modern processed and refined foods end up taking a toll on society, namely:

- The empty excessive calories are harmful and induce fat storage
- They are riddled with artificial ingredients and chemicals that damage our bodies, on both a microscopic and macroscopic level
- Health care costs associated with this Westernized diet are skyrocketing, with obesity predicted by some to be the #1 health care cost in the near future (if we aren't there already)

This trend of overconsumption and its related costs is not sustainable for a healthy society. And when I say not sustainable, I am really sugar coating this and biting my tongue… hard. The only way to improve our health is if we focus on both the quantity we consume, and even more importantly, the quality—that is, foods that are naturally high in nutrients and minerals. In this age of overconsumption of empty calories, that goal may seem unattainable, but I can assure you it is really quite simple.

## Food Building Blocks — Macronutrients

The word macronutrients doesn't mean macro as in a triple cheeseburger. I'm figuring you know that, but surprisingly two-thirds of the population hasn't grasped the true definition. Macronutrients refers to the big three types of nutrients: carbohydrates, fats and proteins. I have tossed fibre in there as an honorable mention, since it is key to a healthy diet.

### Carbohydrates

Carbohydrates are found in foods ranging from spinach to pasta and from beans to cereal. The families of carbohydrates are saccharides (sugars)—mono (one), di (two), and poly-saccharides (many sugars). Carbohydrates are eventually broken down in the body to a mono-saccharide called glucose. This is your body's preferred source of fuel. Although much of the body can burn alternative sources of fuel for energy, the brain and red blood cell production rely on glucose.

Although necessary for energy, as will be explained in detail, excess carbohydrates—the kind you ingest by stuffing your face with that chocolate sundae—elevate your blood sugar and prompt an insulin spike, both of which can become harmful to the body. When eaten with fiber, protein, and fats, carbohydrates absorb more slowly, tempering the insulin response. Managing the secretion of insulin is key to maintaining a healthy lifestyle.

## Fats

Fats are often misunderstood. Contrary to what has been indoctrinated in the public's consciousness since the mid-20th century, fat does not necessarily make you fat. Several studies have shown that even high fat intake does not promote cardiovascular disease or obesity.

One classic study, *The Seven Countries Study* by Ancel Keys, essentially absolved fats of their unsubstantiated link to cardiovascular disease. The study was then handed over to the McGovern committee—a committee formed in the U.S. from 1968–77, tasked with dealing with the rising concern of hunger and malnutrition. For the most part, the committee ignored the findings, maintaining the attack on fats in the media. Despite fats being vilified throughout history, what really has the potential for promoting excess body fat are simple carbs (I'll harp on this throughout).

Fats are a key part of our physiology. Our brains are predominantly made of fat, and our cell membranes are composed of fat. Fat-soluble vitamins, such as vitamins E, A, D and K, need fat in order to be absorbed by our intestinal tract. And hey, it makes a lot of things taste better!

A book could be written on fats alone, but I'll attempt to keep it brief and deliver what you need to know.

There are 3 types of fat:

- saturated
- monounsaturated
- polyunsaturated

A dishonorable mention needs to be given to predominantly man-made trans fats, which I will explain later.

Saturated fats, such as coconut oil and some animal fat, are typically inert and can last a long time in ambient conditions. Monounsaturated fats are simply fats with one double bond (don't worry about the significance of the double bond, we'll just refer to it for identification purposes). Examples of foods with monounsaturated fats are avocados and olive oil. Polyunsaturated fats have more than one double bond. This is where we find our omega-3s—often associated with fish oil—and omega-6s. Let's break these down one by one.

### i. Saturated Fats

Ironically, saturated fats—demonized decades ago, and often supplanted by the much more unhealthy *trans fats*—are actually a necessary component to our diet. You can find saturated fats in several different foods, namely, dairy, meat, and certain oils such as coconut oil.

It baffles me how the public is advised to avoid saturated fats, despite having so many powerful roles in the body. They play a key role in cell membrane function, increase satiety (that "full" feeling), help transport fat-soluble vitamins (A, E, D, and K), and are building blocks for several hormones. Even the heart prefers saturated fats for energy.

Why is it that the public is being told otherwise? Because health claims like these are contrived to protect the interests of food-manufacturing companies. This is why it is so important to do your own research, rather than blindly putting faith in advertising.

It's no surprise that since the advent of the low-fat

craze, cardiovascular disease rates have gone up. Why is this? Because, despite previous studies claiming the opposite, saturated fats in moderate amounts actually help heart health. While I do not advocate excessive saturated fat consumption, recent studies have even shown that being in the high or low range of saturated fat intake has little affect on heart health. (*American Journal of Clinical Nutrition*, March 2010; 91 (3): 535–546).

The much bigger problem occurs when you replace saturated fats with carbohydrates; especially processed and refined carbohydrates, such as starches and sugars. Over-processed grains fit into this category as well, in that they are easily and completely digested, much like sugars. In fact your body can barely tell the difference between most sliced bread and a can of soda. Shortly, I'll elaborate on what happens to your body when you overload on carbohydrates, namely the cycle of insulin resistance, metabolic syndrome (including obesity), and adverse affects on your cholesterol profile.

So let's sum up the saturated fats conversation. While saturated fats are key to a healthy diet, you need to exercise moderation, meaning foods like red meat should not be part of your daily diet, and you should avoid excessive tropical vegetable oils.

Let me leave you with some other advice for consuming saturated fats:

- **Coconut Oil:** Use coconut oil instead of olive oil for cooking, as it has a much higher burning point. When you cook with olive oil at high temperatures it actually oxidizes and develops carcinogenic, cholesterol forming compounds.
- **Organic Butter:** Avoid margarine (contains hydrogenated vegetable oils—trans fats) and substitute it with organic butter. The whole push for margarine in the mid-1900s was misguided. Trans fats have been found to contribute to several diseases, such as cancer and hormone imbalances. (*The Atlantic*, "How Vegetable Oils Replaced Animal Fats In The American Diet, April 26th, 2012)
- **Animal Fats:** These include red meat, chicken, dairy, and eggs. Obviously these all have varying amounts of saturated fat content, with red meat containing the highest concentration. While I do not believe any dairy should be included in a healthy diet, if you do eat it, try making sure it is organic, and preferably raw (unpasteurized). Unfortunately, this is very difficult to find in North America.

### ii. Mono- and Polyunsaturated Fats

Before getting to the star of the show—polyunsaturated fats—let's give a very brief overview of mono-unsaturated fats.

Mono-unsaturated fats are an important part of a healthy diet. You can find large amounts of this fat in red meat, nuts, and fruit high in fat, such as avocados and olives. Mono-unsaturated fats have been shown to reduce LDL (bad) cholesterol, and are therefore good for heart health. Ideally, about 10–15% of your diet should include this beneficial fat.

Last but defintely not least—polyunsaturated fats. When people discuss poly-unsaturated fats they often refer to their star, omega-3s, though omega-6s are another key constituent.

Omega-3s are extremely important fats as they are key for cognitive function, are anti-inflammatory (inflammation—which will be discussed in detail later in the book—can lead to a very extensive list of illnesses and diseases), and help block angiogenesis (the formation of new blood vessels, which is key for cancer growth). The two most important omega-3s are EPA and DHA, while the third omega-3, ALA, garners less attention.

Unfortunately, omega-3s are not prominent in the typical Western diet (also known as SAD, or the Standard American Diet). Fish is a good source but most commercial fish we have access to is laden with mercury. Mercury is a very serious toxin and accumulates in fatty tissue—not great for the brain, to say the least. When possible, choose small wild fish instead, as they are good sources of omega-3s and low in mercury (I've included a handy reference Table in the *Foods To 'Live' By* section). If you choose a supplement, krill oil or other wild cold processed fish oils are good alternatives.

Omega-6s—not only found in whole foods like nuts and seeds, but fast food as well—are overly abundant in our diet. Although necessary in the right quantities, omega-6s can be proflammatory (prompt an inflammatory response), and require higher levels of omega-3 to normalize this effect.

One key point to remember is that omega-3s and omega-6s share the same enzymes needed for conversion. That is why ratios of omega-3s to omega-6s in the range of 1:1 or 1:2 are very important. Unfortunately, however, typical ratios in the Western diet are approximately 1:15. Clearly, we have work to do.

## Cholesterol deserves an honorable mention

The cholesterol we are used to hearing about is in fact a mix of proteins, fatty acids, glycerol, and the molecule cholesterol. Cholesterol is key to proper cell function in that it is necessary for the permeability of the cell wall (important for nutrients entering the cell), and acts as a band-aid for damage that occurs to the arterial wall. It is mainly produced in the liver but also produced in the brain.

Cholesterol has been a hot topic for decades. For the most part it has been misunderstood and vilified as being associated with cardiovascular disease and stroke. In reality, your total cholesterol should not be the predominant indication of potential increased risk for these conditions. The ratio between good (HDL) and bad (LDL) cholesterol is what's truly important. That's what I find incredibly unnerving.

How could all those 'experts' be wrong, you ask? Because that's the crap they were being fed. That's why I call Ikkuma an "evolution". We are continuously muddling through the bullshit claims and rhetoric to find the truth. Problem is, with all the special interest groups, the truth is becoming harder and harder to find.

Since cholesterol is such a hot topic in medical circles, let's investigate high-density lipoprotein (HDL or good cholesterol) and low-density lipoprotein (LDL or bad cholesterol) in a little more detail.

### i. "Good" Cholesterol

High-Density Lipoprotein (HDL): this form of cholesterol simply takes fats and cholesterol from the body and transports it back to the liver for processing. Think of it as a closed system working in conjunction with low-density lipoprotein (LDL).

### ii. "Bad" Cholesterol

Low-Density Lipoprotein (LDL): LDLs are not all bad, as they convey fats (lipids and glycerol) and cholesterol from the liver to the different parts of the body. This process provides fuel and functional elements for proper cell operation. The preferred structure of LDL cholesterol is large and low density, which flows freely through your bloodstream aiding the cells in need. The problem arises with the small, higher density LDLs because they get stuck in the crevices of our damaged arteries, inciting an immune response, which causes further damage and inflammation to the arterial wall. These higher density LDL's typically arise from a diet reliant on processed and refined high carbohydrates.

With all that explained, recent animal research suggests that it is indeed oxidized cholesterol that is the true culprit of inflammation and, effectively, arterial plaque and damage (Staprans I., Rapp J., et al. "Oxidized cholesterol in the diet accelerates the development of aortic atherosclerosis in cholesterol-fed rabits", Jan 1998, *Arteriosclerosis, Thrombosis and Vascular Biology: American Heart Association*). Your arteries are lined with endothelial cells which have receptors that pick up the oxidized cholesterol. Unfortunately, your immune system has bad judgment and recognizes the oxidized cholesterol as bacteria. Macrophages—cells instrumental in defense—are sent to clean up the mess, leaving behind a pile of inflammation.

> ### *Ikkuma* **INFO**
>
> **Free radicals:** We are constantly bombarded with warnings about the detriments of free radicals. Atoms—the building block of any organic element—typically have paired positive and negative electrons. Free radicals are simply atoms with unpaired electrons. They attempt to steal an electron from what they react with. This can be a good or bad thing, depending on the type of free radical and what it reacts with. Due to their reactivity—stealing electrons from other compounds, initiating inflammation—excess amounts of certain free radicals can cause cellular damage and be extremely detrimental to our health. They have been linked to increased risk of cancer, stroke and heart disease. Regarding cancer specifically, free radicals are thought to react with DNA. These reactions can lead to cellular mutations, which begin the chain reaction of cancer. The key is to keep them under control by improving your diet with phytochemicals and antioxidants (effectively neutralizing free radicals), reducing toxins, and dealing with stress (basically everything I will try to help you improve on in this book).

Oxidized cholesterol is the result of overheating vegetable oils (canola, corn, and olive) and mixing them with oxygen. You should not consume overheated vegetables oils at any time. Moreover, most of these oils are derived from genetically modified seeds. The majority of people cook with these oils, not realizing that they have a low burning point and oxidize, which then renders them potentially carcinogenic. So, that extra-virgin olive oil you've been cooking with is possibly doing more harm than heart-healthy goodness. A better choice for cooking is organic coconut oil (a saturated fat), which has a much higher burning point. And remember, you should never be frying at high heat regardless of the oil you are using, because frying at high temperatures can take any oil past its burning point, once again oxidizing the oil.

Here are a few ways to optimize your cholesterol levels:

- Eat a lot of raw food, including healthy fats, such as avocados and heart healthy nuts, such as almonds
- Fiber is key in binding to excess cholesterol before absorption into your system and escorting it out of the body. Load up!
- Consume high quality omega-3 rich fish oils
- Ensure you eat foods rich in plant sterols—organic molecules shown to deter cholesterol absorption—such as nuts and whole grains

- Load your diet with free-radical busting antioxidants, such as kale and blueberries
- Exercise—exercising has been found to help optimize your good to bad cholesterol levels
- Get plenty of safe sun exposure to get rich vitamin D. Vitamin D has been shown to inhibit arterial plaque, offsetting cholesterol's impact

## Protein

Put simply, proteins are the composed of molecules called amino acids. There are twenty-one amino acids in total. Nine of these amino acids are considered "essential", meaning we need them from our food, as the body cannot produce them.

Proteins are building blocks for muscles that perform a number of functions within the body, including factoring in the replication of DNA. There are several different protein sources. Meat is the most commonly known food with a direct association with protein. It is a complete protein source in that its protein has all the amino acids. Most other food has protein as a constituent, but most likely not a complete protein. That is why it is extremely important for vegetarians and vegans to understand what food mixtures will deliver all the amino acids necessary for vibrant health, such as combining beans with grains. Alone they are deficient in certain amino acids, but together they represent a complete protein.

## Fiber

Fiber is an extremely interesting and important part of our diet—which would explain the fiber claims all over boxes of cereal and loaves of bread. What's amazing about fiber is that you actually absorb very little, or none at all—this is exactly what makes it so important. There is no significant calorie intake, yet it provides a vital function in the body. Fiber is classified as either insoluble or soluble. Insoluble fiber, such as the fibrous material in celery, acts as a broom, helping to clean out the intestines, while soluble fiber (examples being found in chia or flax seeds) behaves like a sponge, attracting and absorbing nasty toxins that find their way into the body. It can also aid in the prevention of certain cancers, hemorrhoids and diverticulosis (a disorder which creates cramps and tenderness in the colon). There are several correlations that can be made from the incidence of disease and fiber intake, however one thing is clear: a diet high in dietary fiber is a key component in disease prevention.

# Hormones... The Body's Chemical Messengers

As the title suggests, hormones are the chemical messengers of information throughout the body, critical to ensuring that your body functions without a hitch. Any significant disruption in hormonal balance could wreak havoc on the body. They play roles in everything we do, from telling us when we're hungry or feeling happy, to reproduction. Understanding how key hormones work in our bodies is extremely crucial in truly grasping the effects of foods, stress, and exercise on our bodies.

## Ghrelin/Leptin/Adiponectin/Peptide YY

Ghrelin is a hormone secreted by the stomach. It sounds the alarms that we need to eat, and signals when we need more energy. Conversely, leptin, adiponectin and peptide YY all play a part in letting us know we're full. Specifically, leptin, secreted by fatty tissue, gives us the heads up when we are full and keeps an eye on energy stores; without it we would lose control of our appetite. Adiponectin and peptide YY both sound the alarm, letting us know when we need to stop eating. Peptide YY does this through increasing leptin sensitivity. Note that both proteins and fats are catalysts for the release of peptide YY (PYY), whereas carbohydrates do little to kick start PYY. Hence why we often overeat when our diets are dominated by carbs.

## Insulin/Glucagon

Insulin, probably the most well known hormone, is produced by the pancreas. Its main function is to control our blood sugar levels. You can liken insulin to the 'car' needed to drive glucose (sugar) into our cells. The pancreas goes into insulin-producing overdrive if we binge on simple carbohydrates, as our body processes these sugars very quickly.

Glucagon on the other hand, pulls energy out of yours cells, especially the liver. Glucagon release is stimulated by low blood sugar levels. Insulin drives nutrients into the cell and glucagon drives them out when needed.

## Cortisol

Better known as the stress hormone, cortisol—a key anti-inflammatory—is responsible for a multitude of reactions in the human body. It suppresses immune system "over" response (an overreaction by the immune system), raises blood pressure, and decreases insulin sensitivity. Cortisol can be brought on by external factors, including lack of sleep and stress. As you probably figured out, too much cortisol can be extremely detrimental to good health. It truly is the 'Goldilocks' of hormones—it needs to be just right.

## Insulin-like Growth Factor—1 (IGF-1)

IGF-1 is a big player in physical recovery. Pretty much everything affects IGF-1 release in the body. Yet, excessive IGF-1 can accelerate aging and has been linked to cancer (Cromie W., "Growth Factor Raises Cancer Risk" April 1999, *The Harvard University Gazette*).

Admittedly, this review was a highly simplified explanation regarding hormones, however, for the purposes of this book, it is all that is really required.

# Now It's Feeding Time!

> *"Digestion, of all bodily functions, is the one which exercises the greatest influence on the mental state of an individual."*
> —ANTHELME BRILLAT-SAVARIN, 18TH CENTURY FRENCH WRITER

## Hunger and satiety

I have a tendency to be overly critical of overconsumption. In a world plagued with poverty, it's appalling that

Western society's biggest problem is that we can't control our appetites.

Don't get me wrong. I'm not judging you individually. You may have deep rooted reasons why you rely on food. I'm judging a generation of people obsessed with overconsumption, in every sense of the word. Okay, that's enough barking for now—more to come.

Now that you have a sense of the critical roles certain hormones play in your body, let's dig into how they control your appetite. It all starts with your hypothalamus, where the chemicals for hunger (NPY) and satiety (CART) are housed. The hormone ghrelin gives the signal for you to eat by stimulating NPY, while the hormone leptin stimulates the satiety center (CART) to let you know you should stop. Ghrelin is released by the stomach, while leptin is secreted by fatty tissue.

Things start to fall apart when these hormones stop functioning properly. When people put on weight and consistently overeat, the body becomes increasingly resistant to leptin. You should be able to predict what happens next. If the brain isn't responding to the signal of feeling full, you'll potentially continue eating—leading to a vicious circle of overconsumption. Exacerbating things even further, several foods, such as high fructose corn syrup and other simple carbohydrates, do not prompt the same chemical response of satiety, thus delaying that 'full' feeling. Sticking to diets with a variety of healthy fats, protein, and whole grains will ensure that these signals are heard loud and clear by the brain.

Now that we know why you feel hungry and full, let's look at what happens to the food you in fact do eat.

# Digestion

## Mechanical Digestion... Chewing

Most of you are probably saying, "Why the hell does he think he needs to explain chewing?" We often underestimate how important chewing is to our overall nutrition.

Ironically, we pile more and more food down our throats and probably chew less than ever before. This is a big mistake because chewing stimulates the digestive system to release the appropriate juices—enzymes—it needs to begin chemically and mechanically breaking down the food; this way, the enzymes and chemicals your food encounters later in the digestive process will be able to efficiently break the food down even further. If food isn't properly broken down you will not effectively garner all the nutrients your body needs. In this step of the digestion process, proteins are physically broken down into smaller pieces, the starch component of the carbohydrates and fats are physically and chemically (albeit marginally) altered, and fibers remain intact.

### The Journey Continues... the Stomach

The stomach represents a staging area for food before it enters the intestines. Strong acids and enzymes, such as protein-digesting pepsin, begin digesting your food before moving on to the small intestines. Cells that line the stomach detect food and start sending leptin to the brain to signal that food has arrived, decreasing appetite and increasing metabolism. Fatty tissue in the small intestines will intensify the secretion of leptin. Along with leptin, the stomach releases cholecystokinin (CCK) to initiate downstream digestion.

> *Ikkuma* **INFO**
>
> **Water and meals:** Water is a key to good health and detoxification. As important as it is, drinking at the wrong times can be a detriment to properly digesting our food. When you drink water too close to a meal or during a meal you dilute digestive enzymes and the hydrochloric acid in your stomach. This hydrochloric acid is key to destroying harmful bacteria and it allows the stomach to do its duty of staging food for the small intestines. Aim to avoid water 30 minutes before and 60 minutes after eating, for optimal digestion.

## Intestines

The first stop on our intestinal tract journey is the small intestine. Around the time nutrients enter circulation via the small intestine, the hormone peptide YY is released—the signal that we should slow down our eating by increasing leptin sensitivity. As mentioned earlier, protein and fat help release significant amounts of PYY, with carbs trailing far behind.

Generally, enzymes required for digestion need a relatively hospitable environment. The small intestine is an alkaline environment (this is a good thing), which allows for these enzymes to get busy. With great help from the pancreas in the form of pancreatic enzymes and the gall bladder in the form of bile salts, this is where the true breaking down of our food happens. Complex proteins are broken down into single amino acids, while complex carbohydrates are broken down into mono-saccharides (basically glucose or fructose—essentially sugar). In this state, both get absorbed and enter the bloodstream on the way to the liver. Fats are more complicated. Without boring you with the details (maybe it's already too late for that), fats are dealt with by the bile salts, eventually passing through the intestinal wall. From here, and with the help of special proteins, the fats make their way to the liver, with a few stops along the way.

**SECTION ONE** PART ONE: HOW THE BODY WORKS

## Liver

Did I mention that I used to be a vice-president for an alcohol company? Trust me, you learn to appreciate how important the liver is when you're drinking double vodka sodas like they're water. I can safely say that most of my withdrawals from my Ikkuma Account came in the form of a well mixed cocktail, usually in moderation of course. For this discussion though, we'll discuss the liver as it relates to digestion.

In a **normal feeding state**, broken down proteins (i.e. amino acids) are either used by the liver, converted to other amino acids, converted to sugar, or leave the liver unused. If not used by the liver they are used for dozens of bodily functions, such as muscle synthesis. In times of need, amino acids stored in muscles and other tissues can be used to produce glucose and power the body.

Carbs tell a very different story. When glucose enters the bloodstream post-absorption, the pancreas releases insulin into the bloodstream. The insulin acts as a vehicle, first transporting the sugars to the liver, producing glycogen. Simplified, glycogen is energy stored in your liver and tissues for times of need. The brain and other tissues then use whatever glucose remains as an energy source, if needed.

Things seem fine up to this point—enter fructose. Fructose is a unique carbohydrate in that, essentially, only the liver can use fructose directly. In the liver it is converted to glucose and, as explained earlier, predominatly stored as glycogen.

Lastly, fats simply get transported around the body in the form of fatty acids, performing key cellular functions and are stored to use as future fuel.

There are two main conditions that change the dynamics of how the liver and body deal with proteins, carbs, and fat: a state of *fasting*, and a state of *overconsumption*. In a *fasting* state, the liver tends to convert amino acids (protein) to glucose—sacrificing muscle development—and stores it as glycogen to help maintain blood sugar levels. Carbs get hogged by the liver and saved for optimal brain function and maintaining blood sugar levels. Depending on the severity and duration of the fast, fats get used as fuel through a process called ketosis. Major organs can operate well using ketones for fuel, which helps to reduce the blow to our glycogen stores and muscles.

In a state of *overconsumption*, which seemingly represents approximately 2/3 of the North American population (the approximate proportion of people overweight), things get complicated, and often ugly... very ugly! Proteins do not pose a huge problem. Remember what I said earlier? Protein, through the body's release of PYY, sends a strong signal to the brain that we should stop eating. In the case of excess protein consumption the surplus amino acids are converted to glucose or immediately used for energy.

Here comes the ugly part—carbs. Put quite simply, once the liver and muscles cannot store any more glucose in the form of glycogen, the excess gets converted into fatty acids (palmitic acid) and dropped off throughout the body for fuel, creating loads of fatty tissue.

The greater problem lies in the reaction this fat has with the brain. Constant overconsumption begins to dampen the brain's sensitivity to leptin (the hormone that helps you feel full). Without feeling full, we tend to overeat, and the vicious circle begins. Continuing on this destructive journey, all this excess glucose elevates insulin in your bloodstream and will, over time, decrease the liver's insulin sensitivity and effectively decrease general cell sensitivity to insulin. In effect, your cells become insulin resistant—it takes more and more insulin to get the glucose into the cells that need it. In this state, blood sugar is now getting out of control. Elevated blood sugar starts to create nicks in your arteries—much like sand in a hose—paving the way for an inflammatory response. This inflammatory response is basically the manifestation of your body dealing with the damage that has been created.

As we continue down the rabbit hole, this potential state of insulin resistance starts to trick the body into thinking that it has low blood sugar. You can liken this to a chronic pain you've had for a while. When you begin to experience the pain you are very conscious of it, however after a while you may become used to it. In this situation the body gets used to this elevated state of insulin resistance and it becomes the new status quo. Another way to look at it is through understanding weeds and insects that evolve to adjust to a new herbicide or pesticide. Eventually the invaders evolve and become resistant, requiring more herbicide or pesticide. Similarly, in a state of overconsumption, the body thinks it requires more and more insulin.

Cortisol is the body's next response. Amazingly, despite the saturation of glucose in the body, the body's insulin resistance prompts the production of cortisol, which will work to convert tissue in the body, such as muscle, to glucose. Since muscle is used to store glucose in the first place, the muscle decay amplifies the problem. A good portion of the excess glucose eventually gets converted into fat, and is predominantly deposited around the abdomen. This abdominal fat is not inert. This fatty tissue secretes hormones and molecules that promote dreaded inflammation. Moreover, the fat built up begins to shuttle fatty acids to the organs it surrounds, such as the liver, potentially resulting in conditions such as non-alcoholic fatty-liver disease.

Left unchecked this overconsumption can lead to insulin resistance so severe that a person may develop type II diabetes—a metabolic condition of chronic insulin resistance, characterized by elevated blood sugar.

The last subsequent destructive process in the chain is the production of advanced glycation end products (AGEs). AGEs are formed when all that excess sugar floating around starts to react with proteins in the body and oxidizes. They pose a huge risk due to the mess they make in your body, as they further damage the insulin and leptin receptors (worsening the risk of diabetes), and due to the DNA damage they cause, will accelerate aging.

## I Have a 'Gut' Feeling

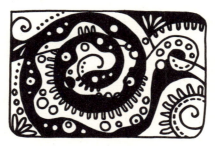

"Vibrant Intestinal Flora"—"The joyful convolutions of life allow us to digest and benefit from the world's abundance."—Sheila LeBlanc

*"It is a hard matter, my fellow citizens, to argue with the belly, since it has no ears."*
—Plutarch, 1st century philosopher

You've heard the expressions, "butterflies in your stomach" and "gut wrenching'". There's a reason why our emotions are often manifested in our gastrointestinal tract, or gut.

You effectively have two brains, one in your skull and one in your gut. Both are created from the same tissue at fetal development; one develops into the central nervous system (in the brain), with the other becoming your enteric nervous system (in the gut), boasting over 100 million neurons. These two systems are connected by the vagus nerve. Therefore, it makes perfect sense that your gut health will have a profound effect on your psychological health. Surprising to many, approximately 90% of the serotonin (happiness hormone) is found in your gut. A happy belly equals a happy person. Your gut is truly the holy grail when it comes to your overall health and happiness. Nuture your gut and your body will thank you for it.

There are trillions of cells in your body, yet, oddly enough, over 90% of the genetic material in your body—not *your* genetic material by the way—is found in the gut in the form of fungi, bacteria (both good and bad) and microflora. This under-appreciated and rarely understood part of your physiology influences your moods, is your portal for getting healthy nutrients to your organs, and represents the majority of your immune system. The gut is the body's first line of defense. It is estimated that up to 80% of your immune system resides in your gut, so once your gut is compromised, all bodily functions, and thus overall health, may be compromised as a result. Unfortunately, few people realize how critical your gut is to how your overall immune system functions.

## What is compromising our gut health?

The following have been shown to destroy your gut flora:

- *Genetically engineered foods:* these foods typically contain higher levels of toxins, which can wreak havoc on gut flora. I'll get into the general GMO (Genetically Modified Organism) discussion shortly. If, after that, you aren't completely disturbed by how far we have let this go, then I have been unsuccessful in laying out the facts.
- *Sucralose:* it has been shown to destroy upwards of 50% of your beneficial bacteria and affects the efficacy of your digestive enzymes (Abou-Donia MB, El-Masry EM, et al. "Splenda Alters Gut

Microflora and Increases Intestinal P-Glycoprotein and Cytochrome P-450 in Male Rats", *J Toxicol Environ Health A. 2008*;71(21):1415-29). I really do think the motto of the 1970s and 80s was how much shit can we invent to trick the public into eating our crap. Just in case you missed my point, sucralose = crap. It shouldn't go near your mouth, let alone in it.

- *Processed foods:* they contain little to no beneficial bacteria, and their typically high level of sugars creates an environment for pathogenic anaerobic bacteria to thrive, thus suppressing good bacteria. These pathogenic microbes damage the integrity of your gut wall. Once the good bacteria has been compromised, it allows the toxins and "bad" bacteria to enter the bloodstream, potentially increasing the risk of developing a host of conditions, including allergies and ADHD.
- *Antibiotics:* this deserves a lot of attention. While there are many different types of antibiotics, all antibiotics kill both good and bad bacteria. While killing the infections they're meant to attack, antibiotics can also destroy beneficial bacteria in your gut. And I'm not just talking about what your doctor prescribes for infection—most people are ingesting antibiotics regularly in their food without

even realizing it. Caged Animal Feed Operations (CAFOs), now a conventional method of raising livestock, routinely use antibiotics to keep the cows, chickens and pigs alive. It's also instrumental in helping animals to grow bigger in a shorter time. Don't even get me started on the animal cruelty. I'd like to be in a room with the sickos who mistreat defenseless animals.

The U.S. FDA reported that over 29 million pounds of antibiotics were used on factory farms. It is estimated that over 80% of all antibiotics used in the U.S. are utilized for some agricultural purpose. But wait, it gets worse. Manure from these operations is laden with antibiotics, contaminating the crops it is used to provide nutrients for. Eventually it makes its way to your stomach, and so the damage begins. What the hell is wrong with us? Our need to pile fast-food burgers down our throats has turned food into a manufacturing business instead of an agricultural one. This is beyond messed up.

When you neglect gut health, the good bacteria (approximately 85% of all bacteria in your gut) is compromised and yeast can grow unabated; literally creating holes in your intestinal lining. This is referred to as leaky gut syndrome, and it can cause a host of problems, such as giving pathogens and other food particles a clear path into the blood stream. Once they get past this first line of defense, these particles are then recognized as invaders, instigating an immune response. This response comes with it a variety of potential complications, namely, allergies and autoimmune disorders.

> ### *Ikkuma* **INFO**
>
> **Know Your Antibiotics:** *The New England Journal of Medicine* found that within the first 5 days of taking azithromycin, a common antibiotic used to treat ailments like ear infections and bronchitis, your chances of dying from heart failure increases by 250%, as compared to taking amoxicillin, another common antibiotic. Know the medicine you are taking. We don't take responsibility for what we put into our bodies. For the few times you really need medicine, it wouldn't hurt to look it up. No excuses!

## Protecting and Repairing Your Gut

Let's look at how you can protect your gut. Hopefully after learning about your gut, you should now realize how critical this part of your physiology is to your overall health.

Here is a quick list of what you can do now to keep it functioning well:

- Avoid the good-bacteria-killing culprits previously listed, with a caveat that antibiotics—medication designed to kill bacteria—should only be taken when entirely necessary. The problem lies with these antibiotics being broad-spectrum (non-specific), as they kill both good and bad bacteria. Good bacteria needs to be nourished, not destroyed. Since non-medical use of antibiotics is not allowed in organic farming, ensure you eat organically raised animals. For beef, look for grass-fed and free-range, and for chickens try to find "pastured" sources.
- Nourishing your gut flora with fermented foods and probiotics is extremely important for brain function—key to regulating your moods. Whole fermented food sources, such as sauerkraut and kimchi, are excellent choices. Organic yogurt, preferably non-dairy, is another good source of beneficial bacteria.
- Control your stress. Later on, I'll give you some tips on how to do that, but know that if you don't control it, your gut health will be but one of the many negative consequences. Stress has been shown to increase the permeability of your gut and be detrimental to your sensitive microflora (P.C. Konturek, T. Brzozowski, S.J. Konturek, "Stress

and the Gut: Pathophysiology, Clinical Consequences, Diagnostic Approach and Treatment Options", *Journal of Physiology and Pharmacology* 2011, 62, 6, 591–599)

# Part *TWO*
## Disease... Know Thy Enemy

*"What can't be cured must be endured."*
—ENGLISH PROVERB

We are currently in the middle of an obesity (now considered a disease!) pandemic, which is contributing to our sky-rocketing incidences of disease; a painfully ironic situation considering we are supposedly one of the most advanced societies in the world. As our wealth grows, so too does our consumption of manufactured crap and fast foods.

As I've already highlighted, the average U.S. citizen's calorie consumption has risen from 2200 to over 2700 in the past 20 years. We are *devolving* into a society that is plagued with *preventable* diseases, as not only are we overconsuming, but what we are eating is often incredibly destructive to our bodies.

What you need to understand is that the way to deal with disease is not only to cure it, but more importantly to prevent it from occurring in the first place. To do this, you need to create an environment within your body that is as conducive to vibrant health as possible—put the focus on prevention!

Don't worry about having a special diet for cancer, and another for diabetes, just be smart with your health. Screw the fad diets and gimmicky get-thin-fast crap out there. Being disease free isn't about short cuts. When will this sink in? As insanely easy as it is to make changes, it's our godlike devotion to the Western diet that is holding us back. But again, don't worry, once you are faced with the reality of your future, unfolding before your eyes, you'll want to change.

Now let's get into a more in-your-face reality; what better topic than disease to brighten up your day.

# Key Precursors to Disease

Before we dive into some common diseases, their impacts, and tips on prevention, let's look at, in detail, two commonly discussed topics inextricably linked to disease: obesity and chronic inflammation.

### i. Obesity

*"My doctor told me to stop having intimate dinners for four. Unless there are three other people."*
—ORSON WELLES, AMERICAN ACTOR

I admit that I used to be a "fat"ist. I'm not proud of it but yes, I judged people harshly based on size. This wasn't because I looked down on them. It was quite the opposite. I just didn't know how people could squander such a beautiful gift as their own health. I have since taken a more empathetic approach and see it as a challenge to help people break the cycle of obesity, regardless of why they ended up obese in the first place.

We've all read studies highlighting the elevated percentages of the population who are overweight and obese. What does this really mean? Remember, overweight refers to having a Body Mass Index (BMI) of 25 or above, while obese refers to a BMI over 30. Out of context these numbers don't really tell you anything. Nonetheless, try checking your BMI (there are several tables on-line to help you with the calculation). If you find you are above 25, then take it as a wake-up call. There is one small caveat, however. If you are very athletic and highly muscular, this measurement is not relevant, and you likely don't even need to be checking your BMI in the first place.

It is estimated that two thirds of North Americans are overweight, and over one-third are obese. As reported in the *USA Today*, if present trends continue, obesity will cost Americans approximately $344 billion in medical related expenses by 2018 (*USA Today*, November 17th,

2009). What's even more disturbing is that over 15% of American children are overweight with another 15% at risk of becoming overweight. Consequently we are seeing skyrocketing rates of type II diabetes in children.

This is one of those, 'Are you fucking kidding me?', moments. How the hell can our children even become an obesity statistic? How can we, as adults, look in the mirror and be ok with this? This isn't about loving yourself regardless of your body type. I see this crap all the time. People encouraged to accept themselves the way they are. Of course we should never be ashamed of our appearance, but this is not about self-esteem. This is about the survival of our children. Stop making this a vanity discussion, because it's not. It's a health discussion. Childhood obesity is not healthy! It's a road to disease and as adults we should be mortified at the simple existence of a childhood obesity statistic.

When discussing obesity, there are two major types of fat we often refer to: visceral (fat that is around your midsection and surrounds your organs), and subcutaneous (just under the skin). Once you have a fat cell, unless you undergo liposuction, you essentially have it for life. It may contract and expand but it will, for all intents and purposes, always be there. It is particularly critical to encourage our youth to adopt healthy habits as early as possible, since most fat cells are typically created by the time we hit puberty.

It's hard to pinpoint the specific cause of an individual's belly fat. Regardless of the reason why you find yourself battling the bulge, visceral or belly fat is a clear sign that your health needs to be refocused. Due to its close proximity to your organs, this type of fat is considered the most dangerous. In order to reduce belly fat, diet should be your main focus, with sleep, stress, and exercise not far behind. While it may not be news to many people, I feel it is important to keep in mind that, in order to successfully fight obesity, it needs to be attacked from every angle.

Although narrowing down your specific reasons for putting on excess fat is tricky at best, cortisol and elevated blood sugar are the most probable culprits in some capacity. Cortisol (the stress hormone), one of the main hormones associated with obesity and the related bad habits leading to it, is released at the end of the dreaded insulin resistance cycle. Yes, we need cortisol to survive, but in excess it eats away at muscle and adds to your visceral (abdominal) fat.

There are several things you can do to keep cortisol from spiking:

- Manage your overall stress, including work, relationships, and so on. Stress can create chronically high levels of cortisol in the body.
- Get adequate sleep. Later on I will outline effective ways to optimize your sleep.
- Avoid excessive sugar and keep blood sugar levels balanced. Sugar comes in many disguises. Don't be fooled! I will drill this home constantly.
- Exercise with purpose. Moderate exercise does wonders to manage cortisol levels.

Elevated blood sugar comes from many different sources, however the process creating this situation is common regardless of the cause. Simply put, eating highly processed, refined carbohydrates will adversely effect your blood sugar. Obviously quantity is a factor, however these foods should be avoided altogether.

Here are some surefire tips to help control your blood sugar intake:

- Eat smaller meals more often.
- Fat, fiber and protein help to regulate the absorption of sugar into the blood, helping to stabilize blood sugar and give you more of that full feeling.
- Reduce refined, simple carbohydrate consumption. This includes high fructose corn syrup (HFCS)—

present in many processed foods—general sugars and overly processed grains, such as those you'll find in white bread and highly refined whole wheat products.
- Eat natural fruits in moderation, in that they contain significant amounts of fructose. However, they also contain vitamins, antioxidants, fiber and other phytonutrients, somewhat offsetting the effects of the fructose.
- When possible, substitute HFCS and sugar with herb stevia or pure dextrose.
- Try to stick with low glycemic foods (see **Ikkuma Info: Glycemic Index**).
- Don't be afraid of fats. Healthy fats such as those found in avocados and fish oil are crucial.

### *Ikkuma* **INFO**

**Glycemic Index:** The glycemic index is a standardized method to measure how much a specific food will increase your blood sugar. The scale is from zero to one hundred. Use the following guidelines to ensure you stick to lower glycemic foods as much as possible:

- High Glycemic Foods (greater than 70) — glucose, corn flakes, white bread, candy, popcorn, baked potato, white bagel, instant oatmeal, soda crackers, watermelon

- **Moderate Glycemic Foods (56–69)** — oatmeal, white rice, whole wheat products, raisins, sugar, sweet potato, corn on the cob, ice cream, spaghetti, honey
- **Low Glycemic Foods (55 or less)** — most fruits and vegetables, whole grain products, brown rice, chicken, meat, eggs, fish, nuts, beans, milk

Many vegetarians contend that they have a much lower chance of becoming obese than those who are carnivores. They support these claims with anecdotal accounts of how slim vegetarians and vegans are, relative to meat eaters. These generalized claims and statements are misplaced, in that being a meat eater means a lot of different things to different people. Eating processed meats and regularly eating red meat, versus eating meat in moderation, are two very different profiles. We need to be careful, then, before placing labels on meat eaters or vegetarians.

I'm not judging vegetarians or vegans. Each to his or her own. Although I'm not a vegan or vegetarian, I do agree that we eat way too much meat. Eating a healthy diet, complete with a variety of whole foods (vegetables and fruit), avoiding refined carbohydrates, and incorporating meat in moderation, is a recipe for avoiding obesity.

Those reading this who are overweight or obese

should not lose hope and submit to the idea that whatever they lose will be gained back. Gaining weight after you lose it is the result of a yo-yo diet. Life isn't about diets. Life and health are about balance. Find your balance. Make some deposits in your Ikkuma Account.

Creating a foundation of good health will help ensure that those pounds stay off. Start today and you'll reap the benefits of weight loss almost immediately. Even minor weight loss can have dramatic effects on your risk of developing chronic diseases. In one study amongst a group of breast cancer survivors, a relatively small 3kg weight loss decreased their risk of recurrence by 24%. (*The Economist*—Dec 15 2012).

Even something as simple as curbing your calorie intake for only 48 hours can reduce fat in the liver by up to 25%. We all need to start somewhere. Set manageable goals and remember that every pound of weight loss counts. A combination of the diet and fitness recommendations in this book can help you begin to eat away at excess body weight almost immediately (see **Ikkuma Info: Intermittent Fasting**).

They key is to make a positive change. Everyone will benefit. Everyone! Trust me, I know it's not easy. I've tried tirelessly to help those close to me, but in the end we all need to find our own motivation.

> ### *Ikkuma* **INFO**
>
> **Intermittent Fasting:** One method some people use to burn fat is intermittent fasting. This could involve an occasional 12–16 hour fast. For instance, on a Wednesday night, have dinner at around 7 pm where instead of eating breakfast on Thursday morning you simply drink water with added pure lemon juice and wait until lunch for your first meal. That would result in a fast of just over 16 hours, helping to expel toxins from your system, while increasing white blood cells (Van Straten, Michael. *Super Detox.*, London: Quadrille, 2003). Moreover, it is theorized that the glycogen stored in the liver and other muscle tissue lasts approximately 8-12 hours before it is used up. After burning these stores the body will resort to burning the most readily available fat stores. That's why eating an early dinner is key. It allows the liver to recover during your sleep, depleting glycogen stores. As an added benefit, when you have your morning workout you are increasingly burning fat for energy.

### ii. Chronic Inflammation

Indirectly, when discussing topics such as gut health and obesity, we have touched on many factors that can lead to what is called chronic inflammation. Inflammation is a natural series of chemical reactions in the body triggered by an abnormal stimulation. This could be caused by something biological, physical, emotional, or chemical.

One simple example of abnormal physical stimulation could be hitting your toe. We all recognize this inflammation as normal and expected; our toe gets swollen, begins to heal, and then returns to normal.

The specific condition of chronic inflammation refers to a state of systemic inflammation brought on by diet (strongly correlated to obesity), stress, pathogens and pollutants, to name a few. It is a state where your body is constantly battling to heal itself—characterized by elevated cortisol levels and adrenal exhaustion. This type of inflammation, left unaddressed, often leads to tissue destruction and a host of diseases.

Due to its involvement in many health problems, this topic will be discussed throughout the book. However, a few examples of specific causes of chronic inflammation should give you a better perspective of how it develops:

- High Sugar Foods: excess blood sugar damages the sensitive lining of our blood vessels, prompting an immune response (inflammation) by the body. This includes using cholesterol, amongst other mechanisms, to repair the vessel lining.
- Acidic Diet: a constantly acidic environment within the body damages tissue, prompting an immune response. Processed foods, refined carbo-

hydrates, and alcohol are guilty of promoting an acidic pH in the body.
- Increased Salt Intake: excess salt intake results in increased water retention in the blood. This increases blood volume, and, in turn, pressure within the vessels. Over time, this will damage the lining of blood vessels, prompting an immune response.
- Chronic Stress: excess cortisol—which, as we now know, is brought on by stress—contributes to insulin resistance due to chronically elevated blood sugar. As seen earlier, this increased blood sugar prompts an immune response.

Those are just a few common examples of how chronic inflammation can be manifested. Once chronic inflammation takes hold, it can lead to several debilitating diseases such as diabetes, cardiovascular disease, cancer, and arthritis.

Let's single out cancer and walk through chronic inflammation's role in its development.

The process starts with chronic inflammation stimulating the immune system, which in turn increases the rate of cell replication. When cells replicate, telomeres within the cell (located at the end of chromosomes), protect them from mutating. Over time, as the rate of replication increases, the length of these telomeres shortens. This exposes the chromosomes to damage, resulting in premature aging and possibly, over time, cancer. This is simply one mechanism; there are several others that come into play for a variety of diseases.

In order to reduce the damage (oxidative stress) caused by chronic inflammation, consumption of antioxidant loaded fruits and vegetables is critical. Here are some other tips to reduce chronic inflammation—note that many of the suggestions in the following list will be explained in detail throughout the book:

- Eliminate sugars and reduce processed and white grain consumption, while focusing on whole, ancient grains. Following a low-glycemic index (low sugar) diet will help maintain healthy insulin levels. Note that the glycemic index, as stated earlier, is simply a standardized measure of how rapidly blood sugar levels rise after consuming a specific food.
- Practice deep breathing. This rids metabolic waste gases through the lungs.
- Avoid trans fats and oxidized cholesterol. Beware of super-heated foods and oils (such as olive oil). Olive oil oxidizes at a much lower temperature, as compared to coconut oil.

- Get your sleep. Sleep helps to relax the nervous system, and allows the body's tissues to recover.
- Ensure a proper omega balance. Ideally, the ratio of omega-6s to omega-3s should be 1:1, rather than the 15:1 ratio typical in today's Western diet (Simopoulos AP., "The Importance of the Ratio of Omega-6/Omega-3 Essential Fatty Acids." Biomed Pharmacother. 2002 Oct; 56(8):365–79). Vegetable oils are a major source of omega-6s.
- Maintain a healthy weight. A more important indicator is the waist to hip ratio. The presence of significant visceral fat is an indication of chronic inflammation
- Exercise regularly. Proper exercise, from walking and restorative yoga, to resistance training and sports, increases oxygenation of tissues through increased blood flow and breathing
- Optimize vitamin D levels, more particularly vitamin D. The best source of vitamin D is through direct exposure to the suns rays. Nature always knows best.
- Reduce stress. Stress causes hypertension, hypertension increases blood pressure, and high blood pressure damages the circulatory system. Stress also increases cortisol levels, damages gut flora, and affects digestion, to name a few.

- Keep hydrated. Acidic metabolic waste that is not eliminated contributes to inflammation. Plenty of pure water helps to alkalize and flush toxins out of your system through the kidneys.

## Common Diseases

Now that the framework has been set regarding the scope of disease's grip on society, and the two main precursors for disease are understood, we can now examine a few of the serious diseases currently rampant in our society, and discuss some tips for preventing them. Before we dive into it, I'd like to touch on a common misconception, namely that genetics plays a predominant role in our risk of developing a major disease.

### Epigenetics

I love how society often uses genetics as a scapegoat for the cause of several diseases. I'm sure you've heard, "My father had colon cancer, so chances are I'll get it to." I'll show you that this just isn't the case. Regardless of your genetics, you play the role of conductor when it comes to allowing diseases to take hold of your body. Stop trying to find lazy excuses and take control. Why dwell on what you can't change? Start doing everything possible to improve what you can change instead.

The field of study related to disease and genetics is called epigenetics. Epigenetics essentially analyzes the correlation between your genetic expression and disease. One famous epigenetic study, *The Human Genome Project*, started in 1990, sought to map out all human genes, and ascertain how to cure or prevent diseases by controlling how genes express themselves. Its initial premise was that information traveled from DNA to proteins, and not vice versa. This, however, is not entirely true. Scientists have determined that the environment—that is, what you think, eat, or are exposed to—effects DNA and how genes express themselves. In other words, it's two-way communication.

This surmises that genes can be activated or deactivated by the environment. I liken it to having one hundred doors (genes), some are locked (no predisposition to a disease) and some aren't (predisposition to a disease). Even if a door is unlocked, unless you choose to walk through it (creating the environment), you obviously have no chance of getting to the other side. That is, the environment that your cells are exposed to, both inside and outside the body, have a considerable effect on how the cells behave. Each cell has a consciousness. Remember, communication flows in both directions.

That means your fate is not necessarily pre-determined by your genetic make-up. You have significant control over your destiny, and over which genes will play a significant role in your health. That is why I am not a proponent of genomic testing for individuals. Learning that you have a predisposition to a certain disease or condition should not necessarily change your habits, as you should already be living the healthiest lifestyle possible. Creating a healthy environment within the body will work to protect you from all disease. Testing only creates unnecessary stress, and we all know that stress can be detrimental to your health.

Nutrition has a direct effect in creating the environment that a cell is exposed to. For instance, we all have tumor suppressing genes and we also have histones, which can effectively neutralize these genes. Cruciferous foods such as broccoli and cabbage act as histone inhibitors, thus allowing the tumor suppressing genes to do their duty of combatting cancers. The more of these foods you eat, the better chance you give yourself of fighting cancer. This is a great example of how diet can control which door you decide to walk through.

A major review on cancer and diet prepared for the U.S. Congress in 1981 estimated that less than 3% of your cancer risk is determined by genetics (Doll R, and Peto R. "The causes of cancer: Quantative estimates of avoidable risks of cancer in the United States today." *J. Natl Cancer Inst 66* (1981): 1162–1265). This is further corroborated by a massive study in China that involved 880 million citizens. It clearly showed that cancer rates among people of the same genetic make-up were significantly different depending on where they lived. Another study by Ken Carroll from the University of Western Ontario showed an extremely strong correlation between a person's geographic location and the diseases they developed (Carroll KK, Braden LM, Bell JA et al. "Fat and cancer." Cancer 58 (1986): 1818–1825). In other words, a person's environment, not genetics, is the main driving force behind diseases such as cancer.

Drop the excuses that genetics grants you. You're only screwing yourself when you dwell on what you can't change. How you treat your body serves as a far more reliable determinant of your future than your genetic make-up. Too many people look for reasons to absolve themselves from the responsibility of managing their health; I am here to tell you that there are no more excuses—your destiny lies almost entirely in your own hands. Proper nutrition, limiting toxins, and positive mental health are the key to having your genes act in a disease fighting capacity.

Understanding that it is mainly us that control our fate, let's dive into some of the key diseases that weigh heavily on society.

## Cancer

Cancer is one word you never want to hear from your doctor. It can be a horrible ordeal. Simply horrible. I lived this first hand with my friend Brad. His suffering was so intense that those of us who were close to him couldn't help but feel his pain. Cancer can be beaten but today's Western diet and associated bad habits are not helping us win the fight. Depressingly, according to www.cancer.org, well over 1 in 3 Americans will be diagnosed with cancer in their lifetime. If you have had cancer or have it now, then I pray that some of the advice in this book may help you.

Our cells are constantly in the cycle of growth (replication), repair, and death. When a cell replicates (mitosis) there is always the opportunity for there to be errors in replication. The more a cell replicates, the more chance for error. Our bodies are supposed to be able to control these errors through a healthy immune system. You probably guessed what comes next. When there are too many abnormal cells and you lose the ability to destroy them at the necessary rate, you develop cancer. That is, your immune system is unable to control the rampant replication of abnormal cells.

This environment of a compromised defense system and increased cell replication can occur with chronic inflammation. Through several hormonal responses, chronic inflammation increases the growth rate of tissues and compromises apoptosis—the process of programmed cell death. If chronic inflammation does not create full blown cancer, as explained earlier, it is still a potential cause of several other degenerative diseases.

Later in the book we will discuss toxins and the several chemicals—called carcinogens—that have been shown to increase cancer rates in mammals. Some you may know very well, such as nitrites (a preservative found in most hot dogs and other processed meats), aflatoxins (originating on moldy corn and peanuts), and some artificial sweeteners.

Now that we've scraped the surface of what cancer is and a few potential causes, let's dig a little deeper into what is exactly happening to the cells in order for them to become cancerous. Cancer has three general phases: mutation, promotion, and progression.

- **Mutation:** most toxins or carcinogens cannot cause cancer on their own. They need to be metabolized (converted) by enzymes in the cell. This new byproduct, called an adduct, then attacks the DNA. If this is not repaired before the cell replicates, you get newly formed mutated daughter cells (cancer cells). Once this happens it is essentially irreversible.

- **Promotiom:** this phase offers a little more hope. Picture the mutation phase as the beginning of a viral video: without other factors to help the video spread throughout the digital world, it would just die an unimpressive death. Cancer behaves similarly: the promotion phase is where your key influencers help spread the material, and allow it to grow uncontrollably. In this phase we start to control our destiny, because without the proper conditions in which to proliferate, such as an acidic environment, cancer cannot overtake the body.
- **Progression:** Once we have reached this stage, where the cancer has metastasized—that is, where the cancer has transferred to another non-adjacent organ or part of the body—we are in real trouble. Imagine weeds coming up through the lawn, and then somehow popping up in your driveway as well. The cancer has spread and has become difficult to contain.

Some studies have shown that reducing the amount of certain proteins in your diet decreases the enzyme activity necessary for binding carcinogens to DNA. The present recommended daily allowance (RDA) for protein is about 10% of our food intake. Most Americans on average consume upwards of 15% of our daily food intake in protein. Some animal studies suggest that this alone, depending on the type of protein, puts us at greater risk of getting cancer (Horio F, Bell RC, et al. "Thermogenesis, low-protein diets, and decreased development of AFB1—induced preneoplastic foci in rat liver." *Nutr Cancer 16* (1991): 31–41).

With that said, further animal studies support the theory that it's not solely the amount of protein, but the types of protein that are relevant. One study in question, analyzing experiments performed on rats, showed that plant-based proteins did not promote cancer growth at levels of 20% protein, where casein protein—found in dairy milk—did (Schulsinger D, Root M, Campbell T. "Effect of dietary protein quality on development of aflatoxin B1—induced hepatic preneoplastic lesions." *J. Natl. Cancer Inst. 81* (1989): 1241–1245). The challenges with dairy will be investigated shortly.

## Common Cancers

### i. Breast

It has been shown that the risk of getting breast cancer is correlated with excessive exposure to estrogen and progesterone. This excessive exposure is typically observed in women who reach puberty at a younger age, and reach menopause later in life.

Studies show that women are indeed maturing

earlier compared to 10-30 years ago (Biro F, Galvez M, Greenspan L, et al., "Pubertal Assessment Method and Baseline Characteristics in a Mixed Longitudinal Study of Girls", *Journal Pediatrics*, Aug 2010). Relative to rural Chinese women, women in the Western world are exposed to over 2.5 times the levels of estrogen (Wu A, Pike M, Stram D. "Meta-analysis: dietary fat intake, serum estrogen levels, and the risk of breast cancer." *Journal Nat. Cancer Institute. 91*(1999): 529–534).

There are many different theories attempting to explain this extension of womens' reproductive lives. As will be explored in further detail later in the book, exposure to many common toxins and chemicals, namely xenoestrogens like phthalates—found in plastics and other household chemicals—disrupt the proper functioning of hormones. Another theory explaining this excessive hormone exposure is linked to our Western diets and habits, which are high in animal protein and refined carbohydrates.

I know I mention excuses a lot. The general public does love excuses, because having one makes us feel free of the responsibility to positively influence our fate. Many people blame genetics as the primary cause for developing breast cancer, and while I won't dispute the fact that genetics do play a role, it's important to qualify how big that role actually is. There are many different studies out there, with one even attributing less than 3% of breast cancer cases to genetics (Colditz G, Willett W, et al. "Family history, age, and risk of breast cancer. Prospective data from the Nurses' Health Study." *JAMA 270* (1993): 338–343).

Even if genetics were to account for two to three times this number, it would still be true to say that a relatively small percentage of breast cancer cases are predetermined by family history. We need to focus on controlling our environment if we want to combat disease. Put the odds in your favor—again, control what goes in your body, control what goes on your body, and control how you keep your body conditioned.

## ii. Prostate/Colon

Rates of colorectal cancer vary greatly from one country to another, with Western societies having the highest incidence of the disease. The argument that environment is a main contributing factor to this disease is supported by many in the field. One report by the World Cancer Research Fund found that rates of colorectal cancer in high-income countries are four times higher than in medium to low-income countries (International Agency for Research on Cancer. *Globocan 2002*). Moreover, many countries that have grown wealthier have seen rates of the disease double since the 1970s (Parkin

DM, Whelan SL, Ferlay J, et al. *Cancer Incidence in Five Continents, Vol.I to VIII*. Lyon: IARC 2005). It is clear that lifestyle, environment and diet, not genetics, are the main contributors towards colorectal disease risk.

Knowing that diet plays a key role in creating that inhospitable environment for colorectal cancer to thrive begs the question, what needs to be fixed? Focusing on increased fiber intake and consuming meat in moderation reduces the risk of developing colorectal cancer. One study's findings showed a reduced risk of nearly 50% when considering these dietary guidelines. (Howe GR, Castelleto R, et al. "Dietary intake of fiber and decreased risk of cancers of the colon and rectum: evidence from the combined analysis of 13 case-controlled studies." *Journal of the National Cancer Institute 84* (1992): 1887–1896). To clarify, by fiber I am talking about natural occurring fiber in fruits, vegetables, and whole grains—not in supplements or fortified food products.

Prostate cancer is a very common cancer, predicted to inflict 28% of American males in 2013 (American Cancer Society, *Cancer Statistics 2013*). While I recommend the same dietary guidelines as above, I stress the importance of also removing dairy from your diet. Increased dairy intake has been shown to double the risk of prostate cancer (Giovannucci E, Chan J. "Dairy products, calcium, and vitamin D and risk of prostate cancer." *Epidemiol. Revs 23* (2001): 87–92).

Again, managing your environment, diet and lifestyle is extremely important in reducing your cancer risk. Cancer is not a natural condition. There are societies and cultures who still eat a predominantly plant based diet and live relatively free of environmental toxins, that have very little incidences of cancer. In the Western world, we continue to rely on modern medicine to combat the disease instead maintaining a healthy diet. Changing from a processed diet to one filled with the phytonutrients—plant nutrients—and antioxidants found in whole foods, will help keep you cancer free.

## Diabetes

Diabetes, specifically type II diabetes (mellitus), wins the award for the trendiest disease in North America. Over 8% of Americans have diabetes, and nearly one third of them don't even know it; our habit of over-eating and heavy reliance on processed and fast food will continue to keep it on the rise.

Before we get into the different types of diabetes, let's quickly review what we have already learned about metabolism:

- after we have eaten a meal, through a series of

reactions in the digestive process, carbohydrates are broken down into simple sugars (glucose)
- the pancreas produces insulin, which is key for getting glucose to our muscles and cells that need it
- the glucose gets used as immediate energy, is stored as glycogen for energy, or is metabolized and stored as fat

**Type I** diabetes is an autoimmune disease where the body's immune system mistakenly attacks healthy insulin producing beta cells of the pancreas. This renders the pancreas incapable of producing insulin. While commonly believed to be genetic, or simply luck of the draw, this is not necessarily the case. Although a genetic predisposition is a factor of the disease, studies have shown that a baby's *environment* is a major factor in the development of the disease. For instance, the introduction of cow's milk to a baby's diet has been linked to development of type I diabetes (Akerblom H, Knip M, et al. "Putative environmental factors and type I diabetes." *Diabetes Metab. Rev. 14*, 31–67 (1998)). There are also studies showing the correlation between a country's per capita dairy consumption and the incidence of Type I diabetes (Dahl-Jorgensen K, Hanssen K, and Joner G. "Relationship between cow's milk consumption and incidence of IDDM in childhood." Diabetes Care 14

(1991): 1081–1083). The stats are even more startling for genetically susceptible children.

*The China Study* (Benbella Books 2006) by Campbell and Campbell clearly explains the process they believe to be behind this phenomenon:

- The baby is fed cow's milk at an early age
- The milk makes its way to the baby's small intestine where the protein is broken down into the individual amino acids
- Some babies are not able to fully digest the cow's milk. In such cases, some of these amino acid fragments can find there way into the infant's bloodstream, and are identified as invaders by the immune system
- The immune system goes about its work destroying these invaders, however some of the fragments look similar to healthy pancreatic cells responsible for producing insulin
- The body loses the ability to distinguish between these fragments and healthy pancreatic cells. The pancreatic cells are then destroyed, leaving the baby with Type I diabetes for life

You can make your own conclusions, though it does seem logical that we should not feed our infants something that has been designed for baby cows. We have evolved over thousands of years, and are designed to nurse our young. If doing otherwise puts our babies at risk, why would we take the chance?

**Type II** diabetes is an entirely different animal. Even though the pancreas is still able to produce insulin, the body no longer responds to it—it has developed a resistance. In other words, your cells—which are used to allowing insulin to feed them with glucose—are so saturated with fats and lipids, that insulin can no longer transfer glucose into them. Essentially the insulin receptors of a cell are desensitized to insulin. Therefore, with the insulin rendered ineffective, the body can no longer metabolize sugars and control blood sugar levels. Liken it to heading to your favorite restaurant, which you have been eating at for years, but because they let in so many tourists, you're now being turned away.

The effects of developing diabetes go well beyond the daily routine of measuring blood sugar levels and taking insulin shots. Diabetes is a disease that opens the door to several other serious complications. Here are just a few, according to the Centers For Disease Control and Prevention. ("National Diabetes Fact Sheet: General Information and National Estimates on Diabetes in the United States, 2000." Atlanta, GA: Centers for Disease Control and Prevention):

- 2–4 times the risk of getting a stroke
- 2–4 times the risk of heart disease
- leading cause of blindness in adults
- leading cause of end stage kidney disease

Once again, the key to dealing with disease is to prevent the disease from developing. Diabetes is no different. You will recognize many of the following tips to avoid developing diabetes, in that they make up a common theme in many "Western Diseases":

- Follow a low glycemic-index diet
- Consume 7–10 servings of vegetables and fruit per day, this will help to alkalize the body, helping to prevent inflammation
- Consume plenty of fiber rich foods, such as beans and legumes, as it helps to reduce cholesterol and maintain healthy elimination of toxins.
- Exercise daily
- Maintain a healthy body weight
- Manage stress levels, as it will reduce cortisol levels and prevent insulin resistance

The sad reality is that type II diabetes is, for the most part, entirely preventable if you adopt a healthy regimen. Therein lies the irony; the one disease we have direct control over is the one that poses the greatest present risk to society. This may as well be the trophy for the generation that overconsumes—our generation. Unfortuntely this trophy has a less than flattering inscription, "To a society that ate itself to death...". This may sound alarmist but when we look back in 20 years, we will be asking ourselves why the hell we didn't wake up when we still had time.

## Cardiovascular Disease and Stroke

Here are some startling facts: nearly 40% of Americans will die from some form of heart or circulatory failure, with women actually eight times more likely to die from heart disease than from breast cancer. (Anderson R. "Deaths: leading causes for 2000." *National Vital Statistics Reports* 50 (16) 2002)

Though the death rate of heart disease has decreased significantly since the 1970s, the actual incidence of it occurring is nearly identical (National Heart, Lung, and Blood Institute. "Morbidity and mortality: 2002 Chart Book on Cardiovascular, Lung, and Blood Diseases." *Bethesda, MD: National Institutes of Health 2002*). This has very little, if anything, to do with an improvement in our quality of life. Instead it is almost entirely due to advances in medical treatment, including the very popular, and far too common, heart bypass surgery. This procedure is a pharmaceutical company's dream, as the patients become heavily dependent on drugs for a prolonged period of time.

As I explained briefly earlier, your absolute cholesterol has little to say about your risk of heart disease; it is your HDL (good cholesterol) to LDL cholesterol (potentially bad cholesterol) ratio that is most relevant. When the endothelial cells lining your arterial walls get damaged—from a poor diet, for example—small and dense LDL particles get stuck and cause inflammation. When this kind of damage occurs, the immune response causes scarring, damage to the blood vessels, and plaque (fatty and greasy deposits) build-up. It is this build-up that restricts flow through the vessels, thus reducing the flow of blood to our vital organs—the beginning of heart disease. From here it can very quickly escalate to a critical level—the artery becomes blocked. Subsequently, the muscles in the heart are starved of the oxygen they need to function. Muscle cells eventually die, kicking off the severe pain and complications of a heart attack. Keeping inflammation at bay is key to reducing the risk of cardiovascular disease, along with a host of other diseases.

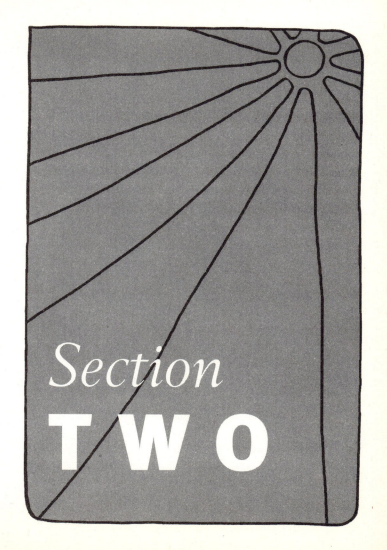

# Part ONE
## Foods To 'Live' By

*(Ikkuma Translation: Feeding The Fire)*

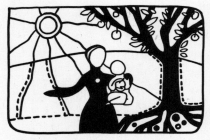

"Nourishment"—"The nourishment that sustains us comes in many places and in many forms."—Sheila LeBlanc

*"We are indeed much more than what we eat, but what we eat can nevertheless help us to be much more than what we are."*
—ADELLE DAVIS, AMERICAN NUTRITIONIST

Okay, so you have a decent handle on how your body works, I hope. While learning how the body works and what causes it to malfunction may have been somewhat overwhelming, it was the basic knowledge necessary in order to truly appreciate the rest of the book. Hopefully you'll read on because in these upcoming sections, I'll focus on foods to incorporate into your diet and why, and foods you should minimize or avoid.

I guarantee that this section, similar to the rest of the book, will spark several "Aha!" moments. Read this and I'm convinced you will change your eating habits tomorrow. That alone is worth the price of admission. A little education goes a long way. It's a lot easier to justify not eating well when you don't know the power of healthy food. Why remain ignorant? In the long run, ignorance only hurts you, no one else.

Unless you're masochistic, I assume you like feeling healthy, energetic and alive. This doesn't happen by accident. Stop being a hero and wake up. You're not superman. We all need good wholesome food… everyday. Yeah, maybe you'll be the one lucky person who eats trash and lives to be 100. Congratulations. Well, the other 99% of people who neglect their nutrition won't be so lucky. Try cleaning up your diet today and maybe making it to 100 years old won't be a fluke. Let's get started!

So, what does our body need? I'm going to dive into this in detail, so let me keep this introduction brief. Essentially our body likes to run on:

- Whole foods filled with antioxidants and phytonutrients, such as a variety of organic vegetables and fruits, to ward off dreaded inflammation
- Whole, ancient grains
- Heart healthy nuts, seeds, beans and legumes
- Fish, eggs and naturally raised meats
- Foods void of pesticides
- Basically anything available during our grandmothers' generation—yes, many of our ancestors did not have access to the same variety of food we have, but what was available didn't have all the adulterants we are now faced with

Overly processed foods are to be avoided. They invariably contain much of what will be vilified later in this section, such as refined sugars and artificial sweeteners. A natural, preferably organic and local diet is key to long lasting, sustainable health.

The majority of individuals get their health and nutritional information from the media—talk shows, television and billboard ads—all sponsored by giant corporations who seemingly lack sincere interest in the public's health. Even more villainous are the ads targeted at children. When I see what food marketing has become, it truly does disgust me. Try watching Saturday morning television with your child and I guarantee you'll be appalled at what we allow companies to push on our children.

It's important to remember that the earth provides us with such an abundance of tasty and nutrient-rich foods that sustaining ourselves on prepackaged products is completely unnecessary. Choose organic produce, legumes and free range, organically fed animal proteins. It's all there for the taking.

While it is important to speak about food, it is also necessary to address one of the most fundamental resources for survival—water. Most of us walking around with symptoms of one ailment or another may very well be chronically dehydrated. In many cases doctors will simply prescribe drinking more water as the first step in a treatment plan for chronic conditions. For example, while water is obviously required for survival, few realize that chronic dehydration leads to increased cortisol production, which introduces a host of other issues.

How much to drink? We've all heard that 8 glasses of water per day (approximately 96 ounces) is sufficient, however that is an extremely crude estimation. A more accurate recommendation is dependent on knowing one's physical activity, size, and other criteria. Roughly, for a physically active 200-pound man, 10–12 glasses should hit the spot. For an average-sized woman, I'd aim for 7–8 glasses per day.

The quality of water is also important to consider. Tap water often contains a plethora of contaminants, including fluoride, chlorine, and hormones. Water filters and water treatment are necessary in order to drink pure, uncontaminated water. There are many options out there but it can be very confusing.

> ### *Ikkuma* **INFO**
>
> **What water is safe? Carbon vs Reverse Osmosis Filtration:**
> There are many options out there to filter the water we drink. I'll touch on a couple of the common ones. First, you have your typical carbon filters, which represent your stand-alone pitcher or a faucet mounted device. Carbon filters chemically bond to contaminants in the water it is filtering. They are effective at reducing contaminants, such as chlorine, lead, mercury and disinfection byproducts; however do not effectively deal with inorganic compounds such as fluoride, arsenic and hexavalent chromium. In many municipalities, though controversial, fluoride is added to the drinking water to ostensibly improve oral health.
>
> Another more involved filtering solution is reverse osmosis. These systems are typically mounted on the counter or under the sink. Reverse osmosis involves passing water through a fine membrane designed to not allow particles larger than water molecules to pass through. It is effective at filtering out both organic and inorganic

compounds. The quality varies greatly from one system to another, however, and they use much more water than they produce. Its use should be limited to cooking and drinking water. There are other systems available, such as water softeners, but for your drinking needs, carbon filters and reverse osmosis are the easiest and most affordable options.

## Key Foods to Eat

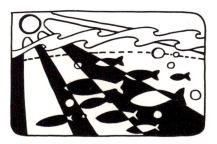

"Living Oceans"—"The vitality of our oceans reflects the level of awareness we are willing to embrace. Let us wake up and work in harmony with the life that seeks to sustain us."

The framework has been set but there are many specific nutritional questions regarding diet yet to be answered. I'll begin by breaking down some key foods to incorporate into your diet, and explain why they are so important for supporting your vitality. This list is not meant to be exhaustive, but simply to highlight the major foods, or food groups. Beyond elaborating on these key foods I will also include some *Ikkuma Top Ten* lists throughout the chapter.

You'll notice that some of these foods are often misunderstood and demonized in the media; the challenge lies in understanding the truth. It's important to scrutinize who is conveying the message and who paid for the related food study, as many are sponsored by multinationals with less than genuine motives. Remember, there are a lot of douche bags out there who could care less about your health. If you don't manage your health, no one will; especially not the multinational food companies.

### i. Eggs

I personally eat about 20 eggs per week. Admittedly this may be high but I just can't get enough. Why am I telling you this? Because eggs are a true super food. They are high in proteins, which, during digestion, get converted by enzymes to peptides, acting as ACE inhibitors—an element common in medications to reduce blood pressure. Eggs have some of the highest levels of biotin in nature; among several other key functions, biotin is key for cell growth. Eggs are also a good source of lecithin, a fatty substance used by every cell in our body, which lowers bad cholesterol. They also contain beta-carotene, which is great for maintaining eye and skin health. The deeper yellow, or yellow-orange the yolk, the higher it is in this important vitamin.

Yes, even the traditionally dreaded yolks are good for you. However, they should be organic to ensure quality, and consumed raw, as the nutrients in the yolks are highly perishable and susceptible to heat. As explained earlier, cholesterol is necessary for every cell in your body, and helps produce vitamin D, cell membranes, and hormones. Studies have actually shown that eggs consumed in moderation have little to no effect on bad cholesterol (*Journal of Nutrition* Nov 1990, 120:11S:1433–1436).

The issue lies with yolks that have been cooked at high temperatures (oxidized), like when you make scrambled eggs. Oxidized cholesterol is directly linked with inflammation which is believed to be a direct cause of cardiovascular disease (Staprans I., Rapp J., et al. "Oxidized cholesterol in the diet accelerates the development of aortic atherosclerosis in cholesterol-fed rabbits", Jan 1998, *Arteriosclerosis, Thrombosis and Vascular Biology: American Heart Association*).

There is a significant difference between commercial eggs and eggs from pastured (allowed to forage for natural food sources) hens. When eggs are naturally raised under sanitary conditions where the chickens are pastured, the potential for salmonella contamination is extremely low. However, due to the disgusting and unsanitary conditions in CAFOs—Caged Animal Feed Operations—the potential for contamination is greatly increased. In 2010, over 500 million eggs were recalled in the U.S. for salmonella contamination that originated from a CAFO. (FDA, *Recall of Shell Eggs*, October 18th, 2010)

Pastured eggs contain less fat and cholesterol, and have higher nutrient levels (e.g. omega-3 fatty acids), as per USDA nutrient data. (Gunnars K., "Pastured vs. Omega-3 vs. Conventional Eggs—What's The Difference?" March 2013, *Authority Nutrition*,) (Karsten HD, Patterson PH, et al. "Vitamins A, E, and Fatty Acid Composition of the Eggs of Caged Hens and Pastured Hens." January 2010, *Cambridge University Press*.) Ironically, eggs that are advertised as having omega-3 should be avoided since they are typically derived from hens who are fed oxidized omega-3 sources. They also typically perish more quickly.

### ii. Meats

I'm not a vegan, nor am I a vegetarian. I find society loves to put people's eating habits in categories. I am of the belief that we have evolved to eat a variety of things on this earth, from meats, fish and eggs, to broccoli and apples. Up until the great agrarian shift over ten thousand years ago, humans ate what was available. I wrote *Ikkuma: Evolution of Vitality* to help us get back to our roots and take advantage of today's variety and availability of great food.

Having said that, I do believe that meat overconsumption is one of the key perils to our planet. The greenhouse gases produced by the meat supply chain is nothing short of mind blowing. If we just cut out fast-food burgers it would do wonders towards solving our climate change problem. *But really Gary, cut out fast-food burgers?* Yeah, I must be insane to even suggest something so stupid.

Though there are many different individual types of meats one could consider, in interest of keeping it simple, my condensed list includes red meat, chicken, pork, and lamb. In order to avoid growth hormones, antibiotics, toxic pesticides and herbicides it is important to always choose free range (preferably pastured) and organically fed meats. With an increase in demand for organic and free range products, these naturally raised meats are now much easier to come by.

An important factor to consider when choosing your organic meat is the saturated fat content (a key inflammatory when consumed in excess), with red meat typically containing the highest levels.

Since discussion of meat tends to gravitate toward the pros and cons—in regards to health—of red meat, I will begin there. While I don't believe red meat to be the enemy, it can adversely affect your health if consumed in excess. What is considered excessive? That's where the confusion begins, since, as with most nutritional advice, there is no clear-cut answer. Remember that we are all unique and, as I will elaborate on when talking about individualized medicine, these differences manifest themselves in a variety of ways depending on the foods we eat. There are studies, however, that can help us make a few general conclusions.

A study published in the *Archives of Internal Medicine* found that life expectancy decreases as meat consumption increases. Many different diseases or "events" were investigated, such as heart disease, cancer and stroke. This study was said to be the first to correlate life expectancy to red meat consumption. It tracked over 120,000 people for 28 years; 20% of the participants died during this period. It was estimated that between 7–19% of those who died would have survived during the study if they substituted one daily serving of red meat with fish or chicken. The final recommendation coming out of the study was to eat 2–3 servings of red meat per week. (CNN, *Too Much Red Meat May Shorten Life Span*, March 12th, 2012). To help control your consumption of red meat, there are many other animal protein sources that can be used as substitutes, including chicken, eggs, fish, pork, lamb and marrow. Saturated fat content varies among these alternative protein sources.

While studies are imperfect—subjects can misrepresent or forget what they ate, and many other factors not being scrutinized can impact the results—they at least give us a starting point upon which to base a decision. Based on what we have been hearing for years, it seems logical that cutting down on red meat would be prudent. Red meat is more difficult for the body to digest and, as mentioned, is high in saturated fats and cholesterol. It is also void of enzymes, which consequently deplete the metabolic, food, and digestive enzymes in our body. Enzymes are critical for food digestion, and help to repair and clean up the inside of our body, so it is important to replenish them by eating raw fruits and vegetables, or by taking an enzyme supplement.

Red meat is also often charred when cooked, producing carcinogens, which contribute to the development of cancer. But with all that said, the real issue is cheap and processed red meat. On top of my earlier rant about the environmental perils, many processed meats are a nightmare to your health, in that they often contain nitrites, believed to promote cancer.

Moreover, unless you are buying grass-fed, naturally raised cattle, you really don't know what's in your meat. In Caged Animal Feed Operations (CAFOs) there can be a host of chemicals in the meat that aren't fit for humans, such as drug residues, heavy metals, e-coli, various antibiotics, and hormones. One alarming fact is that, although antibiotics have been banned in Europe since the 1990's for growth promotion in cattle, most antibiotics are still allowed for growth promotion in the U.S. In fact, in 2009 over 29 million pounds of antibiotics were used on livestock in the U.S. (FDA.gov, 2009 *Summary Report on Antimicrobials Sold or Distributed for Food Producing Animals*).

Despite these arguments, singling out red meat as the culprit to our ills is not the solution. As I'll mention throughout the book, focusing on the overconsumption of refined foods and sugar in the Standard American Diet (SAD) is a more fruitful pursuit in curing the ails of modern Western society.

### iii. Vegetables
If you search for the most nutrient dense food with the least calories, vegetables are where you would end up. Vegetables are critical for our survival. Typically, the

deeper and darker the color, the higher their antioxidant and phytochemical content. Phytochemicals, or phytonutrients, are loaded with the disease fighting antioxidants—critical for battling inflammation and illness. One of the most common groups of phytochemicals are called flavonoids.

Vegetables create an internal force field against several chronic diseases. Starchy root vegetables, like sweet potatoes, should make up about 20% of your vegetable intake. Fibrous vegetables consumption, including the beloved green leafy vegetables, should make up the remaining 80%. Fibrous vegetables have a lower carbohydrate content and are lower on the glycemic index than starchy root vegetables. Cruciferous vegetables from the brassica family, including cabbage, broccoli, and cauliflower, are some of the most powerful cancer-fighting fibrous vegetables.

It is critical that you significantly chew or blend your vegetables. This is because, when they are broken down, their enzymes and phytonutrients are more easily accessible, allowing them to be easily absorbed, and in turn, utilized by the body. This is why smoothies (see Ikkuma Info: Ikkuma "Limitless" Smoothie on the next page) loaded with fresh vegetables are a great idea.

## *Ikkuma* **INFO**

**Ikkuma "Limitless" Smoothie:** I have been experimenting with smoothies for decades. This recipe may seem daunting at first, but it really isn't that hard if you stage all the ingredients. I'll try to make it as clear as possible. First I will list what needs to be staged, and then I will give you the recipe.

To be staged (prepared):

**"Fruit & Vegetable" Mixture:** Clean and chop, beets, apples, purple cabbage, broccoli, celery, ginger, kale and garlic (one clove). You can effectively use whatever vegetables you want but I stress a good variety. Chop enough for about one week's worth of smoothies (use trial and error for this one). My experience is that chopped vegetables, placed in a sealed container with one or two paper towel sheets at the bottom, keep relatively fresh for about one week. This will save a ton of time when making your smoothies.

**"Seeds of Life" Mixture:** Using a coffee grinder, grind sesame, chia, and flax seeds. Place them in a sealable bag and store in your freezer. Try to keep it relatively fresh by only staging two—four weeks worth of the mixture.

**SECTION TWO PART ONE: FOODS TO 'LIVE' BY**

**The recipe:**
Add the following ingredients to your high powered blender and blend until desired consistency:

- ¼ cup of organic almond or coconut milk
- 2 cups of the Fruit & Vegetable mixture already prepared
- 1 heaping tablespoon of the Seeds of Life mixture
- 25–35 grams of high quality natural whey protein (or a vegan protein powder, such as sprouted brown rice, pea, or hemp)—approximately 10 grams less for women
- ½ cup of organic frozen berries and 1 tablespoon of shredded coconut
- 2 heaping tablespoons of organic yogurt (coconut yogurt can be used if you have dairy intolerance)
- ¼ tsp cinnamon to stabilize blood sugar and ¼ tsp of turmeric powder to load it with cancer fighting compounds
- 1 tsp of maca root powder for an energy kick (find this at any health food store)
- 1 heaping teaspoon of glutamine for muscle repair (if desired)
- You can also add a serving of your favorite fish oil
- 2–3 ice cubes (if desired)

One word: AMAZING!! This has incredible body repairing, immune system boosting, gut populating, cancer fighting, age reversing, and antioxidant flooding goodness.

There is a small caveat: if you don't have a VERY powerful blender, vegetables from the brassica (cabbage, broccoli and kale) family may not be fully broken down and promote gas. Try to introduce these vegetables slowly. If they still remain an issue, simply substitute with other fruits or vegetables such as spinach, and avocado.

### IKKUMA'S TOP 10 Vegetables

| Vegetable | Notable Nutrients | Benefits |
| --- | --- | --- |
| Spinach | Vitamin K | • bone health! Activates osteocalcin, promoting calcium to bind inside bones<br>• aids in absorbing vitamin D |
| Onions | Rich in powerful sulfuric compounds and quercetin | • defends against prostate and stomach cancers, and repels osteoclasts (which break down bones)<br>•chopping them helps release enzymes |

| Mushrooms | Selenium, antigen binding lectins, angiogenesis inhibitors, aromatase inhibitors | • antigen binding lectins (stick to abnormal cells, helping the body identify and attack these cells), angiogenesis inhibitors (inhibit the new blood vessels tumors need to supply their energy), aromatase inhibitors (help reduce the production of excess estrogen) — excess estrogen promotes breast cancer |
|---|---|---|
| Kale | Significant in calcium, iron, vitamins A, C and K, and beta-carotene, and loaded with antioxidants | • one of the highest concentrations of antioxidants<br>• incredible cancer fighter and loaded with detoxifying enzymes |
| Sea Vegetables (kelp, wakame, kombu) | Iodine, calcium, iron and all mineral trace elements in the ocean. | • they are alkalizing and help to lower cholesterol (through binding to cholesterol molecules) |
| Celery | High in silica, insoluble fiber | • effective at lowering blood pressure<br>• great for snacking and juicing |

| | | |
|---|---|---|
| Cabbage | Contain indoles and anthocyanins | • part of the brassica family, is a strong cancer fighter |
| Broccoli | High in isothio-cyanates and over a dozen incredible nutrients | • helps in neutralizing carcinogens, it's a cancer fighting all-star |
| Beets | High in bethane and folate | • supports healthy liver function<br>• inhibits homocysteine, which is a contributor to heart disease<br>• good for athletic endurance |
| Brussel Sprouts | Loaded with folate, potassium, sinigin and vitamin K | • strong cancer fighter, leveraging sinigin to promote apoptosis (prompts cancer cells to commit suicide) |

## iv. Fruit

Fruits are similar to vegetables in that they too contain significant amounts of inflammation fighting antioxidants, with the darker colors typically containing the highest concentrations.

The main difference between fruits and vegetables does not lie in their nutritional content, per se, but in their levels of sugar—in the form of fructose. An upcoming section of the book offers an explanation as to why fructose consumption should be scrutinized.

Briefly speaking, fructose spikes insulin, which, as explained earlier, can have significant long-term effects. It also promotes inflammation, and since only the liver can metabolize fructose, excessive amounts can burden it with added stress.

The reason why fruit in its natural form should not be of concern is due to the fiber contained in the fruits. Fiber acts as a regulator for digesting the fructose in the fruit. This is the main difference between fruit juices and whole fruits. Fruit juices allow the fructose to be absorbed much more quickly than in whole food form. This spike may not allow your body to properly use up the fructose before metabolizing it, storing it as fat (Segal M, Johnson R, et al. "How safe is fructose for persons with or without diabetes?", *American Journal of Clinical Nutrition* November 2008, 88(5): 1189–1190). Apart from those who have specific issues like diabetes and metabolic syndrome who should be moderating their consumption of all sugar sources, I would urge you to eat organic fruits as part of a very healthy diet.

It is important to note that since the body digests fruits very quickly, it is preferable to eat them either between meals or before a meal. If not, the fruit will sit in your gastrointestinal tract longer than optimal, and potentially start to rot and ferment in the gut. This could manifest itself as indigestion, heartburn, and other mild reactions. Making this a common habit could potentially cause serious damage to the microflora in your delicate gut.

## IKKUMA'S TOP 10 Fruits

| Fruit | Notable Nutrients | Benefits |
|---|---|---|
| Lemon | Minerals & Vitamin C | • stimulates the liver and digestion, while acting as an efficient detoxifier |
| Pineapple | Bromelain, Vitamin C, trace elements | • supports digestion and reduces inflammation<br>• unlike other fruit, can be eaten after a meal |
| Apples | Various flavonoids (antioxidants) | • helps fight cardiovascular disease and asthma<br>• great for adding sweetness to smoothies |
| Pears | Similar to apples | • high in fiber and a low allergenic potential for those who do not tolerate apples |
| Avocados | High in heart healthy monounsaturated fats | • very versatile for recipes<br>• can be used as a spread for sandwiches |
| Blueberries | Anthocyanin (powerful antioxidant) | • known to protect memory<br>• high antioxidant value, free radical reduction |

| | | |
|---|---|---|
| Cherries | Anthocyanin, quercetin and ellagic acid | • helps support apoptosis (suicide of cancer cells) and has strong anti-inflammatory properties |
| Raspberries | High in fiber, antioxidants and low caloric | • similar to other berries and also fights against cervical and breast cancer |
| Strawberries | Similar to other berries | • works to inhibit cancer's progression, and are good for memory |
| Grapefruit | Low glycemic, Vitamin C | • shown to reduce insulin resistance<br>• warning: causes several medications to stay in system longer (Mann D. "Drugs That Interact With Grapefruit on the Rise", November 2012, *WebMD Health News*) |

### v. Legumes (e.g. Beans)

"Beans, beans the magical fruit, the more we eat the more we toot!" We all remember this rhyme growing up as kids. Yes, beans tend to give us a little gas but beans and other legumes can be a very key aspect of a healthy diet. Legumes contain a mixture of protein, carbohydrates, and loads of fiber. The high fiber content of these foods is key to normalizing cholesterol, stabilizing blood sugars and promoting healthy bowel function. Little do many people know, we should be having as many bowel movements as we do major meals. If you do 'number 2' less than twice per day, maybe you need more beans.

The protein, or amino acid content, in beans is not as complete as that found in animal protein, so we consider it an incomplete protein. When combined with a whole grain, such as brown rice, millet or quinoa, which also contain an incomplete but complementary profile of amino acids, they form a relatively complete protein. This is especially important for vegetarians and vegans, as complete proteins are vital for hormone and neurotransmitter synthesis, muscle repair, immunity, and the many other functions.

Back to the gas, which is, at least to a certain degree, preventable. The source of gas comes from a sugar in the covering of the bean, called oligosaccharides. Since our bodies only absorb about 50% of the bean's carb calories that we eat, there is a lot of fuel leftover to produce gas. Being inherently difficult to digest, these oligosaccharides ferment in the lower intestine—acting as prebiotics—and cause gas. Prebiotics are indigestible foods that act to create more beneficial bacteria in the gastrointestinal tract. Beneficial bacteria equals a healthier gut and a healthier you.

Soaking dried beans in water overnight can reduce

the gas-causing effects of beans. In the morning discard the soaking water, rinse, and cook in fresh water. Another way to decrease this displeasing side effect is to introduce relatively small amounts of more easily digestible beans, such as lentils, mung, adzuki and black beans. The larger beans, such as chickpeas and kidney beans, typically produce more gas.

Looking at other common legumes, I have to begin with a peanut warning—yes, peanuts are legumes. Peanuts can be contaminated with a mold, called aflatoxin, which is carcinogenic. They should not be eaten raw. We are also aware of the growing intolerance to peanuts, so be careful when dealing with these legumes.

Other than peanuts, however, this food family contains an abundance of available nutrition, such as cancer-fighting phytonutrients and polyphenols. As stated in an *American Journal of Epidemiology* study (Singh and Fraser, 1998), which took place over a period of twenty years, people who ate more than two servings of legumes weekly, versus less than one serving, were 47% less likely to develop colon cancer. (Singh, P. N., and Fraser, G. E. (1998) Dietary risk factors for colon cancer in a low-risk population. *American Journal of Epidemiology* 148, 761–774)

## vi. Whole Grains

I argued about grains with Angelina—my ND sounding board—for the longest time. In the end, I conceded and now support the advice that the right grains can be part of a balanced diet. In fact, the carbohydrates within grains are the primary and first choice of fuel for the human body. However, I can't stress enough that not all grains are created equal. Chances are that it is the simple carbohydrates of refined grains—the villians of this story—that are shortchanging your health.

Complex or unrefined grains are preferred, as they contain both the starch (carbohydrates), fiber and germ component of the grain. These components provide our bodies with a more sustainable energy source, along with a lower glycemic load (a lesser effect on increasing blood glucose levels) than refined grains. The whole grain is also more nutrient rich than its refined offspring, containing B vitamins, vitamin E, and many minerals such as magnesium, zinc, iron, as well as calcium and selenium (in select grains).

Fiber consumption is typically extremely low in the Standard American Diet, which is likely a major contributor to many chronic Western conditions like high cholesterol, gall stones, constipation and colon cancer, to name a few.

This is why I—cautiously—emphasize the

importance of including whole grains in your diet. I say cautiously because one must be on the lookout for gluten containing grains, as they can lead to gut inflammation—an important precaution to take, as the rates of gluten intolerance are on the rise. Focus on whole, gluten-free grains such as brown rice, millet, oats, quinoa, amaranth and buckwheat. Common gluten-containing whole grains include whole wheat, barley, spelt and rye.

### vii. Fish

I don't think there is anything that digusts me more than the way we have polluted our waters. Last time I checked, two-thirds of the surface of our precious earth is water. We have somehow—basically in the past two centuries—dumped so much shit in the oceans that we've actually chemically altered the millions and millions of fish we rely on. Think about that for a second. It's appalling and incredibly entitled of us to think we had the right to piss away such a critical natural resource. The fish you eat will never be the same.

Despite how badly we have messed up our oceans, numerous studies have shown that eating 2–3 servings of fish per week is beneficial. Along with having low concentrations of saturated fats, the benefits of eating fish are derived from their high concentration of healthy fats (i.e. omega-3s), protein, and vitamins. Fish can also be great sources of iodine, iron and choline. Put all these anti-inflammatory nutritional powerhouses together and you find a food that lowers the risk of cardiovascular disease, cancer, stroke, diabetes and Alzheimer's.

Sardines and wild Alaskan salmon are especially high in omega-3s with relatively low levels of mercury. Take note that farmed salmon is very different from wild salmon. Farmed salmon can be fed grain, resulting in significantly less heart healthy omega-3s, and more omega-6s in the fish. Moreover, the "net pens" where they are farmed are similar to Caged Animal Feed Operations, except in water. Largely due to the unsanitary conditions in these "net pens", farmed salmon are regularly fed antibiotics to ward off disease. The Environmental Working Group—a leading environmental health research and advocacy organization—found that "an average farmed salmon had 16 times the dioxin-like PCBs found in wild salmon." (EWG, *PCBs in Farmed Salmon*, July 31st, 2003). In restaurants, farmed fish is my biggest concern. Ask the server for clarification if the fish is wild or farmed.

As alluded to earlier, a relevant issue with fish consumption is their concentration of heavy metals, including mercury. Larger and longer living predatory fish will typically have the highest concentration of heavy metals and toxins. These fish eat smaller fish, resulting in the associated toxins accumulating in their fatty tissue. Tuna steaks and swordfish are perfect examples. Regardless of how the fish is prepared, the mercury content will not be affected. Canned white and flaked tuna should also be avoided. Skipjack tuna, which is smaller and much lower in mercury, is preferable. Wild salmon is also relatively low in mercury, especially wild Alaskan salmon.

It is also good to note, that although all fish has mercury, they are also high in selenium, which is a powerful chelator of mercury (helps to neutralize it). You therefore want to stick to fish low in mercury, so that the selenium content can do its magic, allowing you to properly reap all of the other health benefits.

While choosing which fish to eat is not an exact science, it is important to be aware of which types to avoid. See the Table below for a list of some popular fish with relatively high mercury content (Source: FDA):

## (High) Mercury content in various fish

| Fish | Mean Mercury Concentration (ppm) |
| --- | --- |
| Grouper | 0.448 |
| Sablefish | 0.361 |
| Chilean Sea Bass | 0.354 |
| Tuna (canned albacore) | 0.350 |
| Halibut | 0.241 |

| Snapper | 0.166 |
|---|---|
| Perch (freshwater) | 0.150 |
| Tuna (skipjack) | 0.144 |

Since mercury accumulates in fatty tissue there is not necessarily a safe limit, so try to limit the exposure as much as possible. The following table lists some popular fish with relatively low mercury content (Source: FDA):

**(Low) Mercury content in various fish**

| Scallops | 0.003 |
|---|---|
| Salmon (canned) | 0.008 |
| Clams | 0.009 |
| Shrimp | 0.009 |
| Oysters | 0.012 |
| Sardine | 0.013 |
| Tilapia | 0.013 |
| Anchovies | 0.017 |
| Salmon | 0.022 |

### viii. Nuts and seeds

Seeds are the potential for new plant life. Raw nuts and seeds are nutritional powerhouses, packed full of minerals such as magnesium, zinc, potassium, and calcium. Generally high in protein, they are also a good source of healthy fat, and fat-soluble vitamins A, E, D, and K. They are, however, high in fat calories, with each gram of fat containing 9 calories—that's over twice the amount you'll find in proteins and carbohydrates. While they should not be avoided, it is important to be mindful of the amount consumed. Due to their high fat content, some people may find difficulty in digesting them; roasting can amplify this problem.

### *Ikkuma* **INFO**

**Top Digestion Tips:**

1. Eat while you are relaxed and take your time. Being in a relaxed state will optimize digestion. Digestion begins in the mouth, so chew your food well.
2. Avoid drinking water or any liquids while you are eating. Liquids will dilute your digestive juices and lead to gastric reflux, gas, and bloating. Avoid large amounts of liquids at least a half an hour before and after eating. If you need liquid to wash down your food, refer to Tip #1!
3. Eat simple meals and avoid eating large amounts of food at one meal. Simple food combinations promote healthy and efficient digestion. A large amount of food at once slows digestion, which can lead to indigestion and fatigue.
4. Eat fruit on its own, between meals. Fruit digests very quickly and can ferment if eaten after a large meal, leading to gas and bloating.

> 5. Soak beans and legumes to improve their breakdown. Introduce beans and legumes into your diet slowly, and in small amounts.

Although nuts are excellent sources of nutrients, they are also high in omega-6 oils. These oils are necessary for optimal metabolic functioning of the body, however when the ratio of omega-6s to omega-3s is thrown off kilter, trouble can arise. Again, eat nuts in moderation and consume ample sources of omega-3s to keep your body in balance.

## To Be or Not to Be Organic

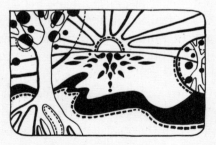

"One World"—Health and vibrancy echos out in a world that knows it's wholeness. We are forever connected to every one and every thing. There is only One World, it is our duty to nurture it.

Let's talk about organic food. Eeeeeks, isn't this a hot topic these days? I can hear your arguments against organic food already. Save it. I can't have a rational argument with people who think chemically doused food is equivalent to naturally cultivated food. *Oh, but studies show that conventionally grown food is nutritionally equivalent.* I'm sorry but I'm calling bullshit on that one. Read on and you tell me.

And don't even get me started on GMO (Genetically Modified Organisms) foods. If chemical companies had nothing to hide then their legal bills wouldn't be greater than the GDP of some small countries. Seriously, wake up. These companies don't spend money for nothing. Anyway, be patient, we'll get to GMOs soon.

I'm encouraged to see that one of the major growth sectors in the food industry is organics. Certified organic foods are produced without the use of synthetic chemical fertilizers and pesticides, are not irradiated, have no chemical food additives, nor do they contain any genetically modified components. Why the hell would you choose otherwise?

There are many Certified Organic regulating bodies that have varied regulatory requirements, some of which are stricter than others. One common and trusted organic certification is USDA Organic.

The majority of people still view organics as a luxury

for the wealthy or an ideology supported by hippies. It's hard to blame the general public for this distorted view of organics, in that they have been inundated with propaganda from the huge chemical companies touting the benefits and safety of conventional farming and the ineffectiveness of organic food.

Please note that we are often sold on the term "natural" as being synomymous with organic. In no way does the term natural imply the same benefits as organic food. The natural claim is highly unregulated, allowing companies to take liberties using the term. Foods that are termed natural can be genetically modified, use synthetic pesticides and contain food additives. In order to get the benefits, you need to buy foods labeled as Certified Organic or better yet, learn the practices of a local farm that follows organic practices.

Before we get into the heart of the organics versus genetically modified organisms conversation let's paint a picture of our existing chemically dependant food supply. The estimated current use of pesticides in the U.S. has surpassed 1 billion pounds per year, or approximately 4 pounds of pesticides per person (M. Rodale, *Organic Manifesto*, Rodale, 2010). Alarmingly, these pesticides are finding their way into our bodies, in that practically everyone has some trace of pesticides in their blood. It is found in amniotic fluid, which means even our babies are being born with pesticides in their blood. (A. Aris, S. Leblanc, "Maternal and fetal exposure to pesticides associated to genetically modified foods in Eastern Townships of Quebec, Canada." *Reprod Toxicol*: May 31: 528–33)

At the heart of this chemical dependancy are genetically modified seeds, used for the majority of conventionally grown foods. These seeds are on the Generally Regarded As Safe (GRAS) list, and considered equivalent to non-GMO. This affords the companies selling these patented seeds the ability to distribute them freely without the necessity of proving long-term safety. As such there have been no long-term studies done on how they affect our health. Chemical companies spend billions of dollars to ensure the government maintains this status quo. They actively lobby against labeling of GMO foods, and dismiss the need for long-term studies. Public awareness on the detriments of GMO terrifies them, because they know that once people become educated on the severe toll their products may take on our health, they will avoid consuming them as much as possible.

To start decoding the organics versus GMO mystery we'll first get into the weeds (excuse the pun) on GMO and then end on a strong note with organics. Sifting through the rhetoric is tricky at best. The focus will be on what we know now and why we should be wary of what we don't know.

## GMOs and Chemical Farming

In the next several pages I'm going to paint a picture using existing studies of why you should be incredibly concerned that GMO foods have become so ubiquituous in today's society.

I'm not some crazy conspiracy theorist. I'm a pragmatic engineer and businessman by trade who has worked for multinational food and beverage companies. I've seen this issue from both sides, and one side is not pretty. We're flipping a coin for our future. We're, for the first time, truly messing with evolution and the delicate interdependancies of all living things.

Just look at the companies controlling this space. Look and ask yourself if these are companies that care about the future of society. I'm sure many of their employees do, but what drives these companies has little to do with the state of the world 20 years from now. Make your own conclusions. I'm personally frightened at what comes next if we don't make it impossible for these companies to stay in business.

## Scope of the epidemic

GMO is an abbreviation for Genetically Modified

Organism. They are organisms that have undergone specific gene manipulation, meaning that specific genes are spliced with certain chemicals or toxins to achieve a desired trait. One common reason for this is to protect certain crops from certain herbicides and pesticides, such as glyphosates.

This agricultural transformation started getting traction back in 1980, when the U.S. Supreme Court, in a close decision, allowed genetically engineered seeds to be patented. This forced farmers to buy their chemical resistant seeds from massive food and chemical companies. 'Roundup Ready' seeds, which survive the abhorrent amounts of pesticides they are subjected to, are the most commonly used chemically resistant seeds.

Following this critical 1980 decision, farming and agriculture would never be the same. What was a fairly natural and family run business was now in the hands of a few incredibly powerful chemical companies.

Three major crops grown with GM seeds are corn, soy and canola. It is estimated that over 75% of all processed food contains GMOs of some sort. In the U.S., it is estimated that approximately 90% of all conventional crops are grown using GM seeds. In addition to the ballooning rates of GM seed use, is the concern of GM crops cross-contaminating (infiltrating) non-GM crops—pollen travels in the wind, so being in close proximity to a GM crop poses a contamination risk. Cross-contamination is an issue because once GM seeds invade a non-GM crop it is very difficult to eliminate this new strain from their fields.

Many farmers don't want to grow GM plants, yet once a crop has been contaminated with the GM seed, not only it is difficult to eradicate the GM seed but they are now beholden to the chemical companies and can be fined if they do not pay for the seed. Without even choosing to use GM seeds, farmers can end up paying giant chemical companies for seeds they didn't want in the first place. I know… unbelievable. Actually unbelivable is too nice a word. This is utter bullshit and shame on the lobbyists who've convinced the government to allow this to happen.

The potential for the approval of GM alfalfa is of special concern because alfalfa is pollinated via insects. This opens the door for cross-contamination of GM and non-GM crops literally hundreds of miles apart. This means that virtually no alfalfa crop will be safe from contamination.

Several European countries—Ireland and Hungary to name a couple—have gone as far as banning the use of genetically modified seeds. It is encouraging that the U.S. principle of "safe until proven unsafe" is not supported by the several countries who are employing a much more precautionary approach.

Companies around the world are also starting to treat GM foods differently from country to country. In the European Union, two of the most high profile companies in the world, Walmart and McDonalds, boast all locations or subsidiaries as GMO-free. They ostensibly do this because, since 1997, the European Union requires labeling of GMO foods, as is stated on the European Commission Health and Consumers website:

> "The EU recognizes the consumers' right to information and labeling as a tool for making an informed choice. Since 1997 Community legislation has made labeling of GM food mandatory for:
>
> - products that consist of GMO or contain GMO;
> - products derived from GMO but no longer containing GMO if there is still DNA or protein resulting from the genetic modification present".

Am I the only one who finds this incredibly hypocritical? These companies brag about being GMO-free, yet in the U.S. where they don't need to label, they freely serve GMO foods. Once again, it's all about making cheap food at all costs. Do you really think they would have stopped serving GMO food in Europe if the labelling requirements hadn't changed?

There are over 50 countries worldwide that require GMO labeling. Amazingly, the U.S. and Canada still do not require any labeling of GMO foods. In the U.S., California drafted Proposition 37, which would have forced companies to label GMO foods—not surprisingly, it wasn't approved. The impetus for the proposition hinged on the belief that if people knew what was in these genetically modified foods, they would most likely choose to avoid them. Companies would then, in order to stay in business, choose to replace these ingredients with healthier, proven alternatives. The powerful chemical company lobby spent millions to defeat the proposition. The increase in food costs became their central defense. Once again, it came down to money.

## The health dangers of GMO and the chemicals involved

While it has been very difficult for scientists to develop a "cause and effect" argument for the impacts of GMO on humans, there are a couple of interesting trends that are important to be aware of: asthma increased by 75% from

1980–1994 (American Academy of Allergy and Asthma Immunology, *Asthma Statistics*) and food allergies have gone up nearly 20% in the last decade (L. Szabo, "Food Allergies in Kids Soar," *USA Today*, Oct. 23, 2008, 7D).

While there very well may be other explanations, we can't dismiss the obvious correlations between the chemical changes in our food chain and the increasing incidences of adverse health conditions. The sad reality is that we don't specifically know what's affecting the health of our children. The reason we have no goddamn clue what is truly causing these trends in children is because they're exposed to soooo much shit. Too many variables exist to allow us to find the culprits. One thing we do know is that without sweeping change, the generations that follow are in for a rough ride.

To give you a sense of what is lurking in your GMO foods, let's look at Bt corn, which represents over 65% of all corn grown in the U.S. Bt corn is the popular corn used in the U.S. that is reisistant to the herbicide Roundup. The protective ingredient inserted into GM Bt corn seeds is Bt toxin. This toxin is inserted in the seeds to destroy rootworms and other insects when consumed. When these insects ingest the Bt toxin their stomachs effectively explode.

It was initially believed that the toxin could not survive in the human stomach, however it is now being found in human blood. In a recent study at the University of Sherbrooke in Quebec, Bt toxin was found in the blood of 93% of pregnant women tested, 80% of the umbilical cord blood, and 67% of non-pregnant women. Clearly, this toxin is not being entirely destroyed in our digestive tract. No one can definitively understand what havoc this toxin is wreaking on our gut flora and immune systems.

Although health issues related to GMOs are relatively unsubstantiated, there is growing research showing their potential links to cancer. One monumental French study found serious links between 'Roundup Ready' crops and large cancerous tumors in rats, as well as damage to several organs. Although this was not a human study it highlights the potential dangers of the consumption of GM foods to mammals (Gucciardi A., "GMO Study: Rats Fed Lifetime of GM Develop Mass Tumors, Die Early." *Natural Society*. 2012 Sept).

Beyond the potential dangers of the GMO crops themselves, there are studies showing the impact of common herbicides used on GMO crops on the human body. A study performed at the University of Caen has found that glyphosates are toxic to human cells (Mesnage R, Bernay B, Seralini GE, *Ethoxylated adjuvants of glyphosate-based herbicides are active principles of human cell toxicity*, Sept 2012). Another study by two Swedish scientists has found a clear link between glyphosates and non-Hodgkin's lymphoma (Hardell L, Eriksson M, "A Case Controlled Study of Non-Hodgkin Lymphoma and Exposure to Pesticides" *Journal of American Cancer Society*, March 15, 1999) . Yet another study has shown that glyphosates also decrease liver enzymes in the body, which then affects the body's ability to detoxify—a vicious circle (Heitanen, et al., *Acta PharmacolToxicol* (Copenhagen), August 1983: 53(2):103–12). Presumably, this is just the tip of the iceberg. Science is shedding more and more light on glyphosates and the potential dangers they pose for humans.

Fearing that consumers become more aware of what's in their food and the related health risks has prompted intense lobbying by major U.S. chemical and biotech firms against the labeling of GM foods. They have been successful thus far, in that there is still no mandatory labeling of GM foods in the U.S. To defeat Proposition 37, in California, it is estimated that the GMO lobby spent tens of millions of dollars to sway the public vote. It obviously worked but who the hell voted against GMO labeling? Over 50% of Californians sided with the chemical companies. That alone should scare you. That alone should open your eyes to how powerful and influential these companies have become.

There are several arguments these lobbies use to

support the use of GMO foods. Let's look at a few and analyze the claims:

- *'Genetically modified organisms are equivalent to non-GMO'*: this argument relies on the fact that seeds have been cross-bred for thousands of years, seemingly without any detrimental effects to humans. GMO is different from cross-breeding. In GMO, toxins, animal genes and bacteria, are being spliced into these new GMO seeds. Therein lies the unpredictability of the GMO seeds: we have yet to witness the long-term effects.
- *'Genetically modified organisms produce better yields'*: this is simply unfounded. It has been demonstrated that organically raised food is more resistant to adverse growing conditions, of which we have experienced plenty in the past several growing years. The practice of growing organically may be more labor intensive, but several studies have shown that organic farming out-produces genetically engineered crops. (Mercola Dr., "You'll Probably Accidentally Eat This Toxic Food Today" 2012 May, http://articles.mercola.com/sites/articles/archive/2012/05/15/california-gmo-panel.aspx)
- *'Genetically modified foods are as nutritious as*

*organically raised crops'*: Although GMO seeds may survive the dousing of pesticides, it does not imply that the plant will be robust and healthy. Fertilizers typically contain forms of phosphates, nitrates and potassium, amongst other inorganic components. If the soil is absent of organic nutrition, and the seeds grow because they simply have the three basic componets required for growth, will they be very nutritious? Will they contain all the nutrients our bodies require to thrive? If you feed your child candy and milk for years, they may grow, but definitely aren't healthy. In the end, it's up to you to decide how you want your body to be sustained. What we do know, regardless of nutritional content, is that they have a higher pesticide content. For example, Roundup contains surfactants that allow it to stick to, and penetrate, the plants it is protecting. Therefore, when we consume these plants we are allowing the imbedded chemicals into our bodies, where they have the potential to cross our blood brain barriers. As use of these chemicals increases, so too does the concentration of them in our bodies .

Truthfully, the long-term effects on human health and the environment of genetically engineered organisms are largely unknown. Scientists admit that it is impossible to understand the long-term effects of an organism when you are splicing it with viruses, bacteria, toxins and various allergenic substances. That being said, we may be creating entirely new toxins and allergens whose potential health effects are real. Is this a risk you are willing to bet your health or that of your child on? The time for half-measures has passed. We need to do what we can to revamp our food chain, and eliminate Genetically Modified Organisms.

> ## *Ikkuma* **INFO**
>
> **Some of the Worst GMO Foods:**
> - Corn—it's estimated that over 85% of the corn produced in the U.S. is Genetically Modified, with the 'Roundup Ready' seeds being responsible for most of the crop. Corn is also one of the more ubiquitous foods in the grocery store, finding itself in most processed foods in the form of high fructose corn syrup. Solid arguments have been made that it is one of the leading causes of obesity.
> - Soy—nearly all soy produced in the U.S. is GMO. Nearly 100 million pounds of glyphosates were used on soybeans.

- Sugar—since 2009 in the U.S. there have been sugar beets designed to resist herbicides.
- Aspartame—along with it increasing the risk of specific neurological issues, such as seizures and anxiety, aspartame is often produced using genetically modified bacteria.
- Papayas—genetically modified papayas have been growing in Hawaii since 1999. Although the European Union does not allow their entry to the market, they are sold in North America.
- Canola—over 90% of canola oil comes from genetically modified rapeseed. Canola can be found in several packaged foods.
- Cotton—cotton oil originating from cotton grown in India and China is particularly harmful.
- Dairy—rBGH (bovine growth hormone) is found in a significant percentage of U.S. dairy cows but banned in over 25 countries. Steer clear!
- Zucchini and Yellow Squash—these vegetables join the ranks of those modified to resist viruses.

## And what about the environment...

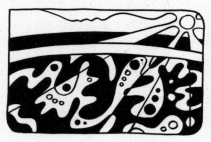

"Soil Dynamics"—The complex life
and vitality beneath our feet is the
foundation for the life and vitality we
seek in our lives. Living soil equals a
vital world.

By now you know that in the U.S., the majority of all conventional crops are born of GMO seeds and that these crops are often doused with the pesticide Roundup. As a result, pests are becoming increasingly resistant to these pesticides, forcing farmers to use more chemicals to get the job done.

A 16-year study published in *Environmental Sciences Europe* found that, although there was a slight dip in herbicide (approx. 2%) use between 1996 –1999, the usage of herbicides spiked sharply due to the emergence of superweeds. These weeds forced farmers to continually scale up their use of herbicides to maintain yields as they had developed a resistance to glyphosates (the active chemical ingredient in the pesticide Roundup). The Environmental Protection Agency (EPA) has also stated that the rootworms may be slowly developing resistance to Roundup Ready seeds (Benbrook C.M., "Impacts of genetically engineered crops on pesticide use in the U.S.—the first sixteen years" 2012, *Environmental Sciences Europe*).

As can be seen in much of nature, organisms may succumb to chemicals in the short term, but evolution catches up and we need to continue scaling up the response. Eventually these pests will be so resilient that even if we were to revert back to traditional methods of control, dealing with them may prove too difficult.

With the need for increasing quantities of chemicals to grow our food, these poisons also find their way into the soil, and can build up over time. The runoff from this soil then enters our waters, which is either used as drinking water, used to water crops—approximately 60% of all fresh water used in the U.S. is used for agriculture (USGS, *Irrigation Water Use*)—or paves a path of destruction in the environment, particularily by compromising aquatic life. In fact, the EPA reported that "more than half of all (U.S.) rivers are unable to sustain life"! Let that one digest for a few minutes! (Associated Press. *More than half of U.S. rivers unable to sustain life, EPA says* March 2013) And reports of the chemicals making their way into our drinking water are not anecdotal. Alarmingly, traces of these chemicals are indeed being found in urine samples (Garber L., "New Study Confirms GMO Crops Causing More Pesticide Use, Superweeds", October, 2012, *Natural Society*).

Chemical farming's impact on the environment doesn't stop at poisoning our soil and water, it can be found everywhere, especially in animals. For instance, due to the extensive use of antibiotics in raising our cattle we are finding newly antibiotic-resistant bacteria in our food. Moreover, the American Academy of Environmental Medicine reports various animal studies showing infertility, accelerated aging, insulin regulation issues, and general organ changes (*American Academy of Environmental Medicine*, "Genetically Modified Foods," May 8th, 2009).

These are not simply observations, they are fact. There are several other animal studies showing causation at many levels between the consumption of GMO foods, and disease in animals. Among them:

- Finamore A, Roselli M, Britti S, et al. Intestinal and peripheral immune response to MON 810 maize ingestion in weaning and old mice. J *Agric. Food Chem.* 2008

- 56(23):11533–11539, Malatesta M, Boraldi F, Annovi G, et al. A long-term study on female mice fed on a genetically modified soybean: effects on liver ageing. *Histochem Cell Biol.* 2008
- 130:96–977, Velimirov A, Binter C, Zentek J. Biological effects of transgenic maize NK603xMON810 fed in long term reproduction studies in mice. *Report-Federal Ministry of Health, Family and Youth.* 2008

Often times when we speak of environmental effects, we speak of the water, soil and animals. We rarely look beyond this, yet one of the most disturbing trends that we are witnessing is the decimation of our honeybee population. This is cause for incredible concern, as Albert Einstein realized in saying, "If the bee disappeared off the face of the earth, man would only have four years left to live."

As discussed in the documentary, *Vanishing of the Bees* directed by Langworthy and Henein, honeybees are crucial for the sustainability of our food supply. They are pollinating workhorses responsible for over 30% of our food supply and pollinate over 100 crops and flowers in the U.S. alone! Other critical byproducts from honeybees' efforts are wax and honey, used for several applications including cosmetics and medicine.

Due to Colony Collapse Disorder (CCD), they are disappearing at an alarming rate. One of the main causes of this phenomenon is believed to be the massive surge of GMO. It is believed that the immune systems of honeybees are being compromised by a new class of insecticides called neonicotinoids. These pesticides get into the soil and groundwater and accumulate, making their way into the plant, including the nectar. Bees ingesting this pesticide have their central nervous systems irreversibly compromised, causing them to die at an alarming rate.

Unfortunately, since it is effective at erradicating insects, virtually all of the genetically engineered Bt corn grown is sprayed with this type of pesticide. Is it a coincidence that honeybee populations starting dwindling after these new pesticides were approved? The European Commission recently imposed a two-year ban on neonicotinoids, citing growing concerns over their effect on the bee population (Woody T. *Honey Bees Are Dying Putting America At Risk Of A Food Disaster*, May 2013, Quartz). Even the EPA admits that pesticides are probably the cause of the dwindling bee population, which we depend on for our food. This is just another reason to avoid GMO and support organic farming. I've read my book at least 200 times and still can't get over some of these facts. I can't believe that we allow these foods to exist.

## Organic farming

I think I've made it pretty clear what I think of GMO foods. And by now, you should have a fairly clear picture of what we're dealing with in regards to GMO and chemical farming. Let's now investigate the state of organic today.

Organic farmland represents less than 1% of the total farmland in the U.S. In Europe this number is approximately 4% (Rodale M., *Organic Manifesto*, 2010 Rodale, pg 149). It's incredibly disappointing and terrifying how little of our land is protected from harmful chemicals. We are far from embracing the sustainable nature of growing organically. In organic farming everything is in symbiosis. Animals eat the plants and fertilize the ground, allowing new plants to flourish. Everything has evolved to work together, without chemicals.

> *Ikkuma* **INFO**
>
> **Earthbound Farms:** Earthbound Farms was founded by Myra Goodman and her husband. With a group consisting of 150 other certified organic farmers, they sell fruits and

> vegetables grown on 33,000 acres of farmland. Without any government subsidies (unlike many conventional farmers who rely on the Farm Bill), they run a profitable business, keeping over 10 million pounds of chemical fertilizers and over 300 thousand pounds of chemical pesticides from contaminating the environment. Lastly, the carbon stored in the healthy, vibrant soil is equivalent to removing 7500 cars from the roads. Can organic farming be viable when it becomes a large scale operation? Earth Farms illustrates that it can.

Let's cut through the negative propaganda from chemical companies regarding organics and look at some results of a Farm Systems Trial run by the Rodale Institute—an American non-profit organization that supports studies in organic farming:

- In times of regular precipitation, organic farming yields are comparable to synthetic methods. However, in times of drought and floods, the deep root structure of organic crops actually produces better yields
- Organic corn and soy crops use approximately 30% less fossil fuels than their GMO counterparts
- Economic return is relatively the same for both methods of farming

- Due to microbials in the soil, there is significant carbon sequestration associated with organic farming. Simply put, while the earth has been designed to store carbon dioxide, the use of chemicals renders it useless.

> *Ikkuma* **INFO**
>
> **Climate Change:** Organically grown crops have very deep and healthy root structures. Mycorrhizal fungi grow on these roots. When present, these fungi sequester carbon in the soil. Unfortunately along with the pesticides, fungicides are often used, which destroy these fungi. It is estimated that if all crops were converted to organic crops, through the great work of these fungi, we would see an instant and significant reduction in our carbon load.

## Organic... The Right Choice

Let's summarize why organic is the choice we should all make:

- Conventional farming is artificially cheaper, in that it's subsidized
- Synthetic chemicals are not necessary
- Chemicals are poison for the soil, food, water, and our bodies

- Chemicals destroy beneficial microbials in our soils
- There is no proven safe limit for toxins
- Organic food is healthier and safer—no antibiotics, no GMO, and no synthetic chemicals
- Organic often tastes better
- Organic can feed the world in a sustainable way—long term

Let's not kid ourselves—chemical farming isn't about feeding the world, it's about making profits. Altruism doesn't increase a chemical company's stock price; uncontrolled chemical farming does. They would have you believe that genetically modified seeds are the saviors of the modern food shortages in underdeveloped countries. This simply is not the case. Tragically, with the advent of GMO and conventional techniques, such as Caged Animal Farm Operations (CAFOs), we have gone down a road that threatens our health, the health of our children, and the survival of our planet.

Chemical industries are not only ignoring the full impact of their products, they have spent the last few decades actively hiding the truth from the public. Millions of dollars each year are spent lobbying for decreased governmental scrutiny, and on funding isolated studies used to convince the public that their chemicals and GMOs are safe for consumption. The fact is, if GMOs were actually safe, these companies wouldn't have to spend so much time and money fighting against GMO labeling. Along with the millions of dollars spent fighting against Proposal 37 in California, another recent example includes a lawsuit threatened by a chemical company on the state of Virginia for a similar proposal.

As Maria Rodale argues in *Organic Manifesto* (Rodale, 2010), the U.S.'s controversial Farm Bill—a federal government food and agricultural policy that is passed every 5 years by the U.S. Congress—creates an even more unfair fight between the defenseless organic movement and huge multinational chemical companies. This $275 billion Farm Bill almost entirely subsidizes the conventional chemical-based method of farming, encouraging the proliferation of GMO. If not for this huge subsidy, and if the total cost of chemical farming were understood—the clean-up of contaminated water, land and soil, and the cost to the health care system—then organic farming would be a more widely accepted long-term option.

The organic movement is all about the long-term view. What goes in the soil gets in the crops, which is eaten by animals, and us, while we then eat the animals as well. Organic farming ensures the quality of the soil is maintained, which means we are getting all of the nutrients from our food that our bodies require. GMO farming typically depletes the soil of nutrition, making plants and animals, and in turn making us, nutrient deficient. Though you may not be able to physically see minerals, nutrients, and phytonutrients, it is important to remember that they are vital for our health and well-being. You may not immediately notice the difference between organic and conventional broccoli, but over time your body will. You might dispute the negative impacts that chemical farming has on the environment but future generations will not have that luxury.

If you could see the chemicals in, and on your food before you ate it, wouldn't you feel differently? We know the right thing to do; yet we convince ourselves that our choices do not have an impact on our health, or the health of our planet.

Despite the overwhelming evidence that GMO food is potentially dangerous to our existence, they are still not adequately tested. Yet another report released in June 2012 by Dr. Michael Antoniou of King's College London School of Medicine in the UK, highlighted that, "Research studies show that genetically modified crops have harmful effects on animals in feeding trials…"— and it goes on.

Since when have we treated our food in terms of

'innocent until proven guilty'? It's time to insist on a change. Don't just talk about it, make changes today. Sadly, due to its ubiquity in our food chain, even if we finally unlock the secrets behind GMO's long term impacts, it would take a monumental effort to reverse the damage.

Bottom line is that it is essentially impossible that organics are not better overall—for our health and the health of the environment. The only argument left is what is your health worth. With only 5.5% of an American household expenditures allocated to food, it's hard to believe that cost is the issue. We spend money on the latest smart phones, eat at expensive restaurants, and enjoy countless other creature comforts, but we convince ourselves that organic food is not worth the extra expense. So, maybe it's an opportunity cost argument, in that if you buy organic food you can't afford the latest electronic gadget. Please. You'll regret it later on. Sadly, it will be too late.

For the fun of it, let's play out the costs. The average in-home spend on food in the U.S. hovers around 5.5%. Let's estimate that the average salary before taxes is approximately $50k. Do some quick math and you'll see that the total cost of food for in-home consumption hovers around $2750. Even if the cost of organic food was 50% more than conventional food (most report it hovering at around 20% more in cost), you're only talking about an extra $1375 per year. Are you willing to play Russian roulette with the health of your whole family for under $1500 per year? That's the true question. Ignore the rest of the rhetoric. Just answer that one question.

Eating wholesome, natural, organic foods is the safest way to go until we know unequivocally that GMO foods are safe for humans and for the environment. Support your local organic farmers. Stop supporting GMOs and huge chemical companies. Demand organic!

## So What About Supplements?

I've talked at length about the good, wholesome foods we should be putting in our bodies for a reason... so you eat them. Don't take this section on supplements as a carte blanche to start shoveling crap down your throat while thinking supplements will fulfill your nutritional needs. They won't. They can, however, serve a few purposes. I'll give you the basics on how to potentially incorporate supplements into your diet.

I define supplements as substances you consume to provide you with the nutrients you may be deficient in, or to give you support in a certain area that needs it. Due to the current state of farming, agriculture and food production, even if we were all doing our best to eat a proper diet, some of us would still require supplementation.

According to a study in *The Journal of the American Medical Association* from 2002, the poor quality of soil is making it increasingly difficult to obtain all your nutrients from diet alone, a reality exacerbated by the fact that significantly less than 5% of our food supply is organic. The majority of the public is not eating properly. According to the U.S. government's survey *Healthy People 2010*, only 3% of Americans eat a meager three servings of vegetables daily. Hence, it is difficult to have all nutritional needs met without some sort of supplementation. Vitamin D is a good example of a nutrient that, unless you get a lot of sunlight, is easy to become deficient in.

Although supplements provide an apparent way out of our nutritional inadequacies, they are not a panacea. Before continuing on to the whole food supplements that could potentially add benefits to your diet, I would like to discuss the little known topic of 'nutritionism'.

## Nutritionism

*"In wilderness I sense the miracle of life, and behind it our scientific accomplishments fade to trivia."*
—CHARLES LINDBERGH, AMERICAN AVIATOR

I turned 41 this year. I was born in the 1970s, during the golden years of the processed food revolution (though, in my opinion, devolution seems a more accurate term). The way we received our nutrition would forever be altered, making the food from our grandparents' era almost alien. The advent of these manufactured food products blatantly disregarded the health of the public for the sake of corporate profits. Population growth was not sufficient enough to satisfy the corporations' desire for profit, so they either had to convince us to eat more or make food a lot cheaper. In the end, both occurred, creating a painful irony; while health claims were used to boost sales, the quality of those products was sacrificed in the interest of lowering selling costs. I know this first hand from my years working for a multinational food company.

Unfortunately, in allowing ourselves to be romanced by attractive packaging, health claims and convenience, we had naïvely given scientists and corporations permission to dictate what was good or bad for us—and we continue to do that to this day. Truthfully, have we made it easy or hard for this to happen? What level of skepticism have you exercised when faced with grandiose health claims? Why do we continue to take things at face value? Have we not yet had the impetus to be even a little bit curious about what goes in our food?

Reductionism was one of the key theories that gave this shift towards fortified foods the nominal credibility it needed. Simply explained, the term reductionism refers to the devaluing of the contextual aspect of an object, relying solely on the characteristics of its parts. As stated by Michael Pollan in his book *In Defense of Food* (Penguin Books, 2008), nutritionism is a form of reductionism in that it defines food as "the sum of their nutrient parts."

In other words, the nutritional value of a food can be measured solely on its individual components (vitamins, minerals, and so on), rather than how those components work together synergistically within the whole food. This application of reductionism is used by food scientists so that they may mechanically recreate specific, appealing components within their manufactured products. Unfortunately, a man-made version of a mineral or vitamin, standing alone, out of context from its original whole food source may never be nutritionally sufficient.

By subscribing to this theory of nutritionism, you are renouncing the relevance of millions of years of evolution—millions of years of nature tweaking the recipe to ensure that organisms were getting the nutrition they needed, not to simply survive, but thrive. Nature didn't design beta carotene capsules, it designed a carrot. The context and delivery system is relevant, and all the interactions and interdependencies between individual food components are relevant.

I liken it to having a beautiful engine in a car but no tires to get anywhere. For the body to absorb nutrients you often need to have certain cofactors and symbiotic nutrients. For instance, you need ample fat to digest fat-soluble nutrients, like vitamin D. In other cases, there are nutrients that simply work better in tandem, such as B6 and magnesium. Studies have even shown cases where, once a nutrient is processed and delivered in supplement form, you no longer reap the benefits. In other cases it may be even be harmful; as seen in preliminary tests where beta carotene increased the growth rate of skin tumors in mice. (National Research Council. *Diet, Nutrition and Cancer*, Washington, D.C.: National Academy Press, 1982: 162–165).

Rather than place value on fruits, vegetables, and legumes, we now value products that are designed and processed from individual components, with claims of every benefit imaginable. Walk through your grocery store's processed foods section. How many products make health claims? How many are fortified with calcium, fiber, omega-3s, or vitamin D? It's dizzying. You need a PhD in biochemistry to pick out a good cereal. And with a marketing budget of over $30 billion annually, U.S. food companies will try to convince you of anything.

Instead of paying for how much it costs to grow and transport your food, you're paying for the convenience and apparent health value that comes from processing and fortification. I say apparent value, because that is exactly what it is. I often harp on the imperfect nature of nutritional science. There truly is no black and white. We don't have nanobots fused to proteins that follow the food as it is absorbed by our bodies. Instead, we have test subjects claiming that they ate this much of this food, at that time, in that proportion. Their information could be biased and inherently imperfect in nature. Even scientists and epidemiologists recognize the severe limitations of the studies they conduct. Health claims are weak at best.

The solution is to simply become more aware. Scrutinize anything that makes a health claim, or better yet, don't buy it. I've been on the other side. I have had arguments with marketers about taking the food out of food and replacing it with cheap garbage. This happened on more than one occasion. Here is a fact for you: companies out there are constantly trying to find new ways to take the good parts of food out and replace them with cheaper fillers that 'mimic' the same nutritional profile. In the end, it's not food. It's a manufactured ingestible substance that has certain designed pseudo-nutritional benefits. Mmmmm, doesn't that sound good? I'll have seconds! Oh, and while you're at it, pass me that turd on the street, as it probably has the same nutritional value as a typical box of cereal.

I can't remember the last time my broccoli had a health claim on it. If it did there definitely wouldn't be a package big enough to do justice to all its amazing benefits. Buy whole foods. Trust in nature. Keep it simple. Leave the turds for the birds. I've been waiting since the second section of the book to insert a 'turd' rhyme. You're welcome.

## Okay, now what?

So when is it a good idea to look into supplementation? Well, the wrong answer is, 'to compensate for a pathetic diet.' I classify acceptable motivations for supplements into three distinct categories: inherent nutritional deficiencies in the food available, environmental influences, and focused performance or health benefit.

Since I've already touched on the nutritional state of our food, let's start with environmental influences supporting supplement use. Environmental influences are grossly underestimated, and an often neglected factor in maintaining our health. People often take the myopic view of environmental influences relating solely to pollution. I classify environmental as any "noise" coming from your surroundings. While this list includes the obvious—exposure to toxins (pollutions) in our air, water and food—it also encompasses stress and improper sleep. Supplements can help deal with these 'uncontrollable' influences in our daily lives.

The last category—focused performance or health benefit—refers to supplementation in order to gain improvements in an area, regardless of diet. Some examples of this could be to improve athletic performance, or to generally bolster energy and stamina.

For as long as vitamins have been around, there has been controversy over their effectiveness. A recent study by the non-profit Cochrane Collaboration—an international network of over 28,000 people in 100 countries, who prepare the largest collection of randomized controlled trials in the world—sheds a little light on this misunderstood subject. It was shown that people, either healthy or sick, had little positive response to taking vitamins A, C, E, beta-carotene or selenium (Bjelakovic G, Nikolova D, et al., *Antioxidant supplements for prevention of mortality in healthy participants and patients with various diseases.* March 2012, Cochrane Collaboration).

There are always many variables to consider, but this does shed light on the inadequacies of specific processed vitamins, further supporting the flaws in reductionism. That is, it is not solely the effect of a micronutrient that is important; it is how it functions in relation to the whole food it is part of.

The common attitude is to simply take a multi-vitamin. This is often a futile endeavor. Again, over-processing takes what nature designed and reduces it to an unnatural form that the body hasn't been designed to ingest. Several studies have even shown that specific vitamin therapy may exacerbate cancers of the breast and prostate.

Vitamins should not be the answer to a poor diet. The answer to a poor diet is to improve it. I'm not saying that vitamins do not have their place, as whole food supplements can be helpful at providing you with specific nutrients you may otherwise be lacking.

Let's take a look at some of my favorite supplements that are often times difficult to obtain in our Western diet.

### i. Omega-3

A typical North American diet includes only a fraction of what the World Health Organization recommends as being the minimum daily intake of omega-3. There are three types of omega-3 fatty acids, namely EPA, DHA and ALA. Omega-3s are essential in that they are necessary for maintaining good health, but the body cannot produce them (EPA and DHA can be produced by the body if you have ALA present, but this is not optimal). Omega-3s are some of the most intensely studied supplements. There are several substantiated claims that supplementing omega-3s is key to preventing several diseases and improving overall health—which is likely due to their anti-inflammatory benefits.

Here is a taste of the impressive resume of omega-3s and why they draw so much attention:

- Reduce brain and cardiovascular inflammation
- Improve cellular health, including skin health
- Optimize fetal brain development
- Support overall brain function, including mood
- Improve glucose and insulin metabolism

Omega-3 fatty acids are typically found in marine (eg. fish) and plant (eg. flax seed) oils. There are many excellent supplements out there. Try to find quality sources that are cold processed and derived from wild, low mercury sources.

### ii. Vitamin D

For several years now vitamin D has been getting significant press for its cancer-fighting and anti-aging properties. There have been dozens of studies regarding recommended doses. It has been shown to reduce chronic inflammation in the body, as well as ameliorate the deterioration of your DNA over time. It does this by inhibiting the body's inflammatory response. In doing this, turnover of cells is decreased, slowing the rate of DNA chromosome telomere deterioration—in turn slowing the aging process and protecting against many diseases, such as cancer.

Getting high quality sun exposure is an extremely efficient way to bolster your vitamin D stores. While we have been sold on how the sun can increase our risk of skin cancer, the chemicals in the majority of suntan lotions—like oxybenzone and parabens—can arguably pose a greater risk to getting cancer than getting safe sun exposure (I'll discuss that in more detail in the section on Toxins).

We are being taught to fear the sun, yet the sun is literally a key to life. Humans evolved to be in harmony with the sun. Our bodies need sun. Yes, there are damaging UVB and UVA rays, however, in moderation, exposure can be healthy.

One little known fact is that midday sun has highest concentration of vitamin D-inducing UVB rays. Yes, you read that right. Start with limited exposure to ensure you do not burn—approximately 15 minutes—and slowly extend the time as tolerance increases. If getting ample sun is not an option, there are high quality vitamin D supplements derived from wild fish oils.

### iii. Chlorella
Chlorella is a fresh water single-celled algae loaded with vitamins, minerals, several trace elements and is rich in chlorophyll. Chlorophyll has an amazing list of benefits:

- Optimizes oxygen delivery to your cells, through increased red blood cell production—more oxygen means more cellular energy
- Through reducing inflammation and supporting good bacteria growth in your intestines, it plays a huge part in bolstering your immune system

Chlorella delivers another often-overlooked nutrient called iodine. Iodine is necessary for an efficiently functioning thyroid. The thyroid gland is a critical factor in hormonal balance and operation. If your thyroid doesn't get the iodine it needs, your metabolism will suffer and your energy levels will decrease. This is why you often hear of weight gain associated with an improperly functioning thyroid.

Like most algae, chlorella is also an effective detoxifying agent, binding to heavy metals and other toxins in the body. Next time you decide to drink more than you should, take in some chlorella to help avoid a hangover.

There are several different chlorella supplements on the market. Look for organic broken-cell-wall chlorella—the cell wall of chlorella is not digestible, so it needs to be "broken" to allow for its full benefits to be realized.

### iv. Resveratrol

Resveratrol is the active compound in red wine that has been getting accolades as of late. Recent studies have touted its anti-aging effects due to its impact on genes related to aging. Regardless of these potential effects, we know that it is a powerful antioxidant that has been linked to:

- Reduced risk of many cancers
- Lower incidence of cardiovascular disease
- Anti-aging
- Bolstered immune system

### v. Magnesium

Magnesium is the fourth most abundant element on earth, and magnesium ions are essential to all living things. Approximately 65% percent is stored in our bones and teeth, and the remaining is found in the blood, fluids, and tissues of the body. It is important for the functioning of hundreds of enzymes in your body, and also plays a key role in interacting with ATP (the energy 'currency' of our cells), RNA and DNA. Since it cannot penetrate cell membranes, magnesium ions need to be paired with transport proteins in supplemental form (chelates).

While magnesium is critical for our survival, it is estimated that over 50% of the population is deficient. This is alarming as it is required for nerve and muscle function, bone health, and regulation of blood sugar. In addition, caffeine, sugar and alcohol cause us to actually lose magnesium, while low acidity in the gut also decreases magnesium absorption.

Magnesium deficiency can lead to several diseases, including diabetes, anxiety disorders, and cardiovascular disease. If you eat a variety of nuts, fruits and vegetables, you shouldn't need to take magnesium supplements.

### vi. CoQ10 (Ubiquinol)

CoQ10 is an essential vitamin used by every cell in your body. It is key to cellular respiration, and generates energy through ATP production—approximately 95% of our energy is derived through this process. CoQ10 is instrumental in offsetting aging, in that it recycles other antioxidants, thus reducing DNA damage.

Deficiency in CoQ10 can cause heart failure, muscle weakness, fatigue, and obviously, pre-mature aging. The older you become the less efficient your body becomes at metabolizing CoQ10. Although it is found in several foods, its ubiquitous benefits in the body have made it one of the more popular supplements in the U.S. Taking a ubiquinol (fully broken down CoQ10) supplement will help offset the difficulty in metabolizing CoQ10 as you age. Moreover, if you are on statin drugs it is advised to supplement CoQ10, as statins deplete CoQ10.

### vii. Astaxanthin

Astaxanthin is an up-and-comer in a powerful class of antioxidants. It's a free radical scavenging beast. Believed to be the most powerful carotenoid—an organic pigment found in plants—it is over 50 times more powerful than vitamin C and beta-carotene (another carotenoid), and over 10 times more powerful than vitamin E at dealing with free radicals (Moerck Dr. *Astaxanthin & key carotenoids: creating leading edge eye healthcare formulations*, Valensa 2013). It also goes to work in areas like the brain and eyes, where certain other antioxidants cannot access, aiding in the protection of your nervous system and sight.

Moreover, while other antioxidants can be overused,

astaxanthin does not act as a pro-oxidant—causing oxidation—even in extremely high doses. Another interesting characteristic of this powerful antioxidant is that is soluble in both fat, and water—meaning it can cross the blood brain barrier, and assimilate in both fats and water in the body, allowing it penetrate and protect the entire cell. As an added bonus, supplementation with astaxanthin can actually act an internal sunscreen. Some great food sources of this antioxidant are krill and other crustaceans, while the oil is available in capsules.

### viii. Vitamin $B_{12}$

$B_{12}$, often known as the energy vitamin, is a key nutrient that we're finding increasingly difficult to obtain within the average diet. $B_{12}$ has been shown to be effective at:

- Repairing and maintaining a healthy nervous system
- Supporting the immune system
- Producing red blood cells
- Sustaining energy levels
- Maintaining cell growth and repair
- Honing mental alertness
- Converting carbohydrates and fatty acids into glucose (fuel)

$B_{12}$ deficiency can be caused by ineffective absorption, or not obtaining sufficient amounts from your diet. It is especially difficult to absorb due to its physical size. Moreover, people with poor diets, over a period of time, can significantly compromise their gut lining. This can become critical, in that parietal cells in the stomach lining produce hydrochloric acid and intrinsic factor—the vehicles for $B_{12}$ absorption.

Apart from animal sources, there are virtually no other effective sources of vitamin $B_{12}$ (the $B_{12}$ in spirulina is an analogue, which is not effective). Even conventional red meat has less and less $B_{12}$, as Caged Animal Feed Operations (CAFOs) restrict any grazing that allows the animals to naturally ingest $B_{12}$ from the grass and dirt.

Summed up, it's becoming increasingly difficult to obtain $B_{12}$ from a healthy diet. Virtually everyone could benefit from supplementing $B_{12}$. When taking a specific B supplement it is important to take it within a whole-food complex as well, as high levels of one B vitamin can actually mask a deficiency of another (eg. a deficiency in $B_{12}$ can be masked by high levels of $B_6$).

There are fantastic organic, whole-food B-complex supplements on the market. We need approximately .4–2.8 micrograms of $B_{12}$ daily, and a typical person has the ability to store 2–5 milligrams.

### ix. Whey Protein

As explained earlier, protein is critical for several basic physiological processes. It is the building block for hormones, neurotransmitters and antibodies, and is crucial for building strong bones and muscles.

Whey protein is a common protein obtained from whey—a byproduct of dairy production. Whey protein has many benefits:

- Easily assimilates in the body for efficient protein supply
- Known as one of the best sources for obtaining the nutrients needed to produce glutathione (incredibly valuable antioxidant)
- Necessary for the formation of white blood cells, which is important for overall immune responsiveness

There are several things you should look for when sourcing whey protein. The critical ones are:

- Whey isolates can be over-processed, so choose a micro filtered source if possible (acid processing potentially denatures the amino acids), such as whey concentrate, which has a beneficial effect in stabilizing blood sugar

- Whey typically contains lactose, so is not appropriate for those with lactose intolerance or a dairy sensitivity. There are lactose free sources.
- It should be derived from hormone-free cows which are grass fed and naturally raised (100% New Zealand whey is a great source, preferably organic)
- It should be cold processed/filtered—excessive heat damages micronutrients
- Avoid products that have artificial sweeteners
- Whey should be free of toxic heavy metals

## x. Probiotics

I've already explained the vital nature of gut health and the importance of re-seeding good bacteria. Neither can be underestimated. The typical Western diet—saturated with high fructose corn syrup, antibiotics, lack of fiber and overconsumption of dairy products—constantly bombards the lining of your gut, posing a significant threat to its health. I would like to point out now that to be proactive and help avoid the stresses on your gut, you should load up on soluble (dissolves in the body) fiber, and plenty of fruits, vegetables, and legumes, which act as prebiotics—substances that promote the growth of good bacteria in the gastrointestinal tract.

As explained, the gut is estimated to be responsible

for greater than 80% of your immune system. The health of your gut flora has a direct effect on your immune system and the quality of your immune response to invaders. Once the lining of your gut is compromised, you may start absorbing improperly digested foods—"leaky gut." This condition allows toxic substances (pathogenic bacteria and viruses flourish in an unhealthy gut) to enter the bloodstream, where some then cling to certain proteins, inciting an immune response. Symptoms of this condition include depression, anxiety, rashes, or abdominal pain.

The key is to heal the damaged gut lining with fermented foods and other probiotics. They are the most effective way to protect and replenish the good bacteria in your intestinal tract. Examples of fermented foods are sauerkraut, kimchi, and cultured dairy products. These cultured foods are also great chelators—or detoxifiers—that help rid your body of heavy metals and other toxins.

While I recommend everyone include fermented foods in their diet, it is especially important for those with leaky gut. Just be sure to introduce them slowly, because if detoxification occurs too quickly you can have a healing crisis, and experience flu-like symptoms. You can start a simple protocol, such as beginning with one teaspoon of fermented vegetables, wait a day or two, gauge your response and continue increasing the portions.

You can also buy probiotics off the shelf. There are literally hundreds of different options out there. Industry standards dictate that you should seek probiotics with at least $10^8$–$10^{10}$ CFU (colony-forming units)/day. CFU is a measure of the active bacterial content in a probiotic.

## Eat Your Power Foods

Superfoods, or, as I prefer to call them, power foods, have become a hot topic. These foods are typically low calorie, yet very dense in nutrients or phytochemicals (plant chemicals). Blueberries or acai are the most commonly known.

Let's take a look at turmeric—a super-spice—in detail, followed by the rest of Ikkuma's Top Eight Power Foods.

### Tumeric powder

Tumeric has been known as a miracle spice in the Eastern hemisphere for ages. In the Western world we are just beginning to understand the benefits of its active ingredient, curcumin. Curcumin is a potent anti-inflammatory agent—loaded with antioxidants—and has documented liver protection properties. It also has impressive immune boosting properties; having been shown to halt certain cancers, and actually prompt cancer cells to destroy themselves—a process called apoptoisis. It does this through influencing dozens of pathways in the cell.

You need to start introducing this into your diet. Of all the power foods you'll find, turmeric is safe and its incredible cancer-fighting benefits are supported by extensive literature. Tumeric can be bought in grocery stores as a spice, or in health food stores as a supplement. Just make sure that it's certified organic and free of fillers.

## IKKUMA'S TOP 8 POWER FOODS

| Power-Food | Benefits |
| --- | --- |
| Tumeric | • See above |
| Nettle | • Due to its high chlorophyll content, nettle is a good source of cellular energy<br>• It is also loaded with iron and several other trace elements |
| Ginger | • Indian medicine recognizes ginger as the "universal remedy"<br>• It is a potent anti-inflammatory, helps with nausea and boosts immunity |
| Cinnamon | • It boasts a newly discovered class of phytochemicals called chalcone polymers, which increase glucose metabolism in cells—blood sugar regulation properties<br>• Shown to lower blood pressure |

| Garlic | • Has been studied extensively for its wide range of health benefits<br>• Anti-hypertensive, antioxidant, anti-microbial, anti-viral and anti-parasitic |
|---|---|
| Sauerkraut & Kimchi | • Effective at re-populating gut with "good" bacteria, which, as explained earlier, improves immunity and digestion<br>• Known to many as some of the healthiest foods, with all the properties of cabbage and more! |
| Bee Pollen | • Incredibly nutritious with almost all known enzymes, minerals, trace elements and amino acids<br>• One of the few sources of $B_{12}$ |
| Spirulina (micro-algae) — could also be considered a supplement like Chlorella | • Great detoxifier — cell walls bind to heavy metals<br>• High in protein, Omega-3s, and 9 amino acids — unfortunately the $B_{12}$ is an "analogue" which does not provide the benefits of the $B_{12}$ you find in meats |

## Alkaline Versus Acidic Foods... WTF? (What's the Fuss?)

Our bodies are a chemical laboratory. One of the indicators of our chemical balance, pH, is the measurement of the acidity and alkalinity of a solution. Our bodies work most effectively at a pH around 7.4, which is slightly alkaline (7 is neutral). If our pH is consistently below 7—a state of acidosis (an acidic environment)—chronic inflammation can occur. As we have learned, chronic inflammation can lead to many degenerative diseases, such as cancer and osteoporosis.

An acidic environment in the body results in leaching of alkalizing minerals from the largest reserve in our body—the bones. Minerals from the bones are used to buffer the blood from acidity, and excess minerals end up being deposited into tissues. Interestingly enough, the Western world consumes the highest amounts of dairy, yet we have some of the highest rates of osteoporosis! This is an example of an acidity issue, not a lack of calcium issue.

In the next major section of the book we will discuss potentially harmful foods in detail. Many of the foods we will discuss are also foods that promote an acidic environment or are acid forming within the body, such as sugar, refined grains, meat, coffee, and alcohol. Don't get confused with the actual pH of some foods and their effects in the body. Although lemon has a relatively low pH—well under 7—it has strong alkalizing effects in the body.

**Acidic forming & Alkalizing foods**

| More acidic | Less Acidic | Types of Food | Less Alkaline | More Alkaline |
|---|---|---|---|---|
| Navy beans, pinto beans | Cooked spinach, kidney beans, string beans | Vegetables/Beans | Peas, carrots, tomatoes, cabage, olives, mushrooms | Onions, raw spinach, broccoli, vegetable juices, garlic, |
| Blackberries, cranberries | Oranges, processed fruit juices, plums | Fruits | Bananas, pineapple, peaches, avocados | Lemon, lime, grapefruit, watermelon |
| Artificial sweeteners | Refined sugar, molasses | Sweeteners | Raw honey, maple syrup | Stevia |
| White flour, pasta, white rice | Wheat, brown rice, spelt | Grains | Amaranth, quinoa, wild rice | |

| Peanuts, walnuts | Sunflower seeds, pumpkin seeds | **Nuts & Seeds** | Chestnuts | Almonds |
|---|---|---|---|---|
|  | Corn oil | **Oils** | Canola oil | Olive oil |
| Beef, pork, shellfish | Turkey, chicken, cold-water fish | **Meats** |  |  |
| Cheese, homogenized milk, ice cream | Eggs, yogurt, cottage cheese | **Eggs/ Dairy** | Whey, Goat cheese, goat milk |  |
| Alcohol, soft drinks | Coffee, tea | **Beverages** | Green tea | Herbal teas, lemon water |

*From www.phreshproducts.com*

While there are also healthy foods that can be acid forming in the body, it is the amount consumed that determines the effect they will have. The key is to balance acidic foods with eating high quality, organic, alkalizing foods, such as kale, raw spinach, almonds and avocados. Fresh vegetable juices, greens powders, such as chlorella and spirulina, and lemon water taken between meals, are great ways to quickly alkalize the body. A good practice to follow would be to eat alkalizing foods for 65%–80% of your diet, with the remaining one third being quality acidic foods, such as eggs and lean meats.

Before wrapping up *Foods To 'Live' By* I'd like to stress that our bodies have evolved over thousands of years, and that this evolution was based on what was available. Our bodies crave real food. It's as simple as that. When you are eating chemically altered and overly processed industrial food, you are essentially eating dead food. Your body needs nutrients, which it cannot effectively get from manufactured foods. Dependence on sugars and processed food is literally like a drug addiction. It may be tough at first to improve your diet, but within days your body will start to repair itself, and within weeks your addiction to modern processed food will fade.

### *Ikkuma* **INFO**

**Typical day of eating and great snack ideas:**

Now that you are armed with a wealth of information regarding what you should be eating, here is what I would consider a healthy day in the life of an Ikkuma inspired eater:

**Morning:** Wake up to a filtered glass of water containing the juice from half a lemon. Immediately drink another glass of water to further hydrate and wash the acid from your teeth. Wait about 30–45 minutes for your metabolism to kick start, and prepare an *Ikkuma 'Limitless' Smoothie* (see recipe earlier in the section).

**Mid-Morning:** If you start to get hunger pangs before lunch, what you need is some healthy protein, fiber and fats to cut your cravings. The following are some great snacks:

| | |
|---|---|
| • Celery stalks w/ almond butter and raisins | • Carrots with hummus |
| • Apple with a hand full of almonds (raw or roasted) | • Kale chips |
| • Organic yogurt (can source coconut yogurt if lactose deficient) and organic blueberries | • Left over vegetables and chicken or fish from the night before |
| • Various berries (low sugar and high fiber) | REMEMBER: YOU CAN'T EAT JUNK FOOD IF IT ISN'T IS YOUR HOUSE! DON'T HAVE IT AROUND! |

**Lunch:** A good option would be a salad with a variety of greens and other healthy fruits and vegetables, topped off with pastured chicken or wild Alaskan salmon. This can be seasoned with balsamic vinaigrette. Quinoa can also be a great addition to the salad.

**Mid-Afternoon:** Always pay attention to drinking water throughout the day. You want to ideally space water consumption at least 30 minutes before or after a meal, in that water consumption during a meal rushes digestion and dilutes critical stomach acids, sabotaging proper digestion. When the need strikes to have a snack in the afternoon, the choices listed for mid-morning are excellent choices at this time of day as well.

**Dinner:** Ideally dinner would be eaten at around 6pm to allow the liver to recover during your sleep. Eating too late in the evening does not allow your liver to get much of a break—after digesting dinner—before it has to get back to work in the morning. A reasonable dinner could consist of some pastured chicken or fish, coupled with a variety of brightly colored vegetables. Starches, such as potatoes, should be limited late in the day. Sweet potatoes or wild brown rice in moderation would be fine for an early dinner.

### Ikkuma Top *Foods To 'Live' By* Tweets:

- Many of us walk around chronically dehydrated. **Water** is the first step to getting healthy. **Find pure sources or use reverse osmosis.**
- **Eggs** are a nearly perfect protein and high in beta-carotene—helps keep eyes healthy. **Pastured eggs are best.** http://bit.ly/13UyB3R

- **Avoid harmful antibiotics and hormones!** Choose organically raised meats. They may also have higher level of critical vitamin $B_{12}$.
- **Load up on green leafy vegetables.** They are cancer-fighters and loaded with antioxidants poised to reduce chronic inflammation in the body.
- **Make breakfast smart!** Load up on low-glycemic, high in fiber foods. My morning **Ikkuma 'Limitless' Smoothie** is a great kick-start to the day!
- **Eat a wide range of colors**. Colorful **fruits and vegetables** are loaded with flavonoids (powerful antioxidants). The darker the better!
- **Stick to high fiber complex carbs,** like vegetables and **whole grains.** The quality fiber helps control the rate of sugar absorption.
- **Smaller fish** like sardines and krill are loaded with heart healthy omega-3s. Ensure supplements are high quality. http://bit.ly/11ukq8m
- **Snack on nuts!** They're loaded with healthy omega-3s and -6s. Nuts also curb your appetite before a meal. Buy raw nuts & lightly roast.
- **Eat while you are relaxed** and take your time. Being relaxed will optimize digestion. Digestion begins in the mouth, so chew your food well.
- **Avoid drinking any liquids while you are eating.** Liquids will dilute your digestive juices and can lead to gastric reflux, gas, & bloating.

- **Eat simple meals.** Avoid eating large amounts of food at one meal. It slows digestion, which can lead to indigestion and fatigue.
- **Eat fruit on its own,** between meals. Fruit digests very quickly and can ferment if eaten after a large meal, leading to gas and bloating.
- **Organic is simply better** for you and the environment. Less pesticides and chemicals in your food can't be bad! http://bit.ly/18CsgwW
- **Steer clear of GMOs.** GMOs are not effectively tested and their properties are potentially harmful http://bit.ly/17fWRBr
- **Vitamin D** has been heralded as a supreme cancer fighter. **Embrace the sun in moderation** for the best source nature has to offer!
- **Go green! Chlorella** is an algae efficient at detoxification and ultra-rich in nutrients. Don't forget that they are great for hangovers!
- **Magnesium is critical.** Deficiency can lead to several diseases. Get it from a variety of dark fruits & vegetables, and nuts & seeds.
- Every cell in the body uses the "energy" vitamin **CoQ10**. It has key anti-aging properties. We need more as we age.
- The king of the B vitamins, yet the most elusive, **vitamin $B_{12}$** factors in cell growth and repair. Organic meats are good sources.

- Upwards of 80% of your immune system lies in your gut. **Probiotics** keep the gut healthy. Fermented foods and yogurt are great sources.
- **Tumeric** needs to be part of your diet! It's a miracle Indian spice that you can find almost anywhere and fights cancer like none other.
- **Load up on alkaline foods.** An acidic environment in the body leads to inflammation & disease. Here are some choices http://bit.ly/18E8AJ3
- **Throw away junk food snacks!** You can't eat what you don't have. Stockpile healthy, delicious, protein & fiber filled options.

## Bonus Ikkuma *Foods To 'Live' By* Tweets:

- **Drink organic green tea.** Its powerful polyphenols help protect your heart and fight cancer.
- **Coffee in moderation can be healthy.** It is a bitter herb that helps detoxify the body and has healthy antioxidants. A light roast is best.
- **Olive oil and cooking don't mix.** A better cooking option, coconut oil, has a higher burning point. Olive oil is best eaten raw.
- **Eat whole foods!** When foods are processed and refined, nutrients are removed from the food, and left out or reintroduced ineffectively.

# *Part* **TWO**
## Foods To 'Drive By'

**(Ikkuma Translation: The Fire Is Starting to Fade)**

> *"Preserving health by too severe a rule is a worrisome malady."*
> —FRANCOIS DUC DE LA ROCHEFOUCAULD,
> 17TH CENTURY FRENCH AUTHOR

"Are you fucking kidding me?" That was my first reaction when someone I was coaching said she didn't want to give up pizza because she liked it. I couldn't believe what I was hearing. Don't get me wrong. I like pizza, and it can be made healthy. But quite frankly I've earned it. I have made a shitload of deposits in my Ikkuma Account. Remember that? It was way back in the prologue to this book. Judging by that formula, your typical pizza is one withdrawal I can make. But if your Ikkuma account looks like a compulsive shopper's credit card, then sorry, no pizza for you—at least not for now.

This chapter is the easiest one to abide by because all you need to do is avoid eating shit that's not good for you. That's it. No sit-ups. No marathons. Just avoid shit. Avoid the shit we invented 50 years ago to make companies more money. Avoid the shit that not even rats should eat. This chapter is easy. Check this box off as done or don't even pretend you want to get healthy.

To make it even easier, I'll give you a piece of advice that will change your life forever. Just don't have crap in your kitchen. If it's not there, you can't eat it. You don't think after a long night out I wouldn't be tempted to eat a bowl of greasy, salty chips? Of course I would. After a couple of cocktails even I can be seduced by the short-term satisfaction of so-called comfort foods.

Throughout the book I attempt to paint a balanced picture of foods and not be too exclusionary. I want to make changes doable and sustainable. Nobody is perfect, yet we can constantly stress about eating perfectly. There are some foods, however, that you really need to avoid. In this section I'll discuss them and encourage you to seriously consider eliminating them from your diet. The key is to make the transition to optimal health manageable within the framework of your already hectic life.

At first you may make excuses on why you can't eliminate or cut down on a certain food. Try to make it easier on yourself by having very short-term milestones. Your body will eventually wean itself from the addiction of these harmful foods and reward you for it. Trust me!

Before I get into the specific harmful food offenders, I want to once again bring to light our global obsession with processed foods. Here are some startling facts, as reported in a December, 2012 issue of the *Economist*:

- 25 million Americans visit McDonalds every day.
- During the past decade alone, the sales of packaged foods have risen by 92%. Soft drink sales have doubled over the same time period.
- In India, Brazil and China, the numbers are even scarier, with soft drinks sales increasing by 400% over the past decade.

Nearly every processed food contains refined grains, sugars, additives, artificial colors and flavors—all of which harm your health. Sadly, in the face of the obesity epidemic, at a time when we should be improving our dietary habits, we are actually digressing at an exponential rate. Let's take a look at some of the food dangers out there.

## Key foods to avoid

### i. Wheat

Estimates are that wheat has been around for at least 12,000 years. With the advent of wheat, ancient civilizations were able to thrive, as it was easy to cultivate, and be stored for times in need. If the wheat we typically eat today was anywhere near the form of ancient wheat, then it may have been spared from this section.

Over thousands of years wheat has undergone tens of thousands of hybridizations, and some is of course, now genetically modified (yet not approved). The result of these alterations has resulted in structural mutations, including increased levels of gluten. Gluten is inherently difficult to digest, and is responsible for some autoimmune conditions, including celiac disease. Another example of wheat's evolution can be witnessed in its protein content, with modern wheat made up of about 15% protein—that's half the content of ancient grains. Unfortunately, truly ancient strains of wheat are next to impossible to find.

The issues don't end there. It has been observed that upwards of 5% of the proteins of wheat hybrids are unique (i.e. not present in either of the parents). These unexpected genetic arrangements may change the protein structures, thus affecting organs in unknown ways. In effect, our bodies are dealing with them for the first time. GMOs creates similarly unique proteins.

There is no real good news here. Fifty years of hybridized wheat has resulted in new strains that our bodies are not adapted to dealing with. Modern wheat also has higher levels of Amylopectin A, which is very easy to digest, and thus spikes blood sugar. Conversely, legumes, like beans, contain Amylopectin B and C, which aren't as easily digested.

Now, you may think that you're making a healthy choice by opting for whole wheat breads, but it, too, is so over-processed and refined that it actually spikes your blood sugar in the same fashion as white bread. To put it into perspective, two slices of whole wheat bread spikes blood sugar to similar levels of a can of soda pop or chocolate bar. This blood sugar high typically lasts about two hours before the crash hits, and this isn't just a sugar high. The polypeptides from wheat, and other carbohydrates, have actually been shown to bind to opiate receptors—meaning wheat has a potentially neurological or addictive effect, stemming from the release of serotonin.

Another comfort food, pasta, spikes blood sugar for 4–6 hours (depending on the variety), though whole wheat pasta does have a marginally muted impact. The reason for the difference in this spike, is due to the fact that pasta is actually metabolized differently than bread. So although you may be consuming a similar amount of carbs, they get absorbed at a different rate.

Never neglect the detriments that spiking blood sugar can have on the body. Remember the vicious cycle: excess glucose—high blood sugar—insulin response—fat—insulin resistance—diabetes. One of the more obvious results of this death spiral is visceral fat. It's unfortunate that what was once such a reliable food staple has been mutated into something that actually contributes to excess weight and health issues.

Now let's get back to the well-known elephant in the room—gluten. As mentioned, gluten is a notoriously problematic protein found in wheat, rye, and other grains. The lectins in wheat, which are rich in proline—a non-essential amino acid—can also cause potential damage to your gut. The issues caused by gluten and lectins are quite similar, in that they both affect the body's immune system, and—similar to dairy proteins—are both difficult for your body to digest.

Once damaged by poor diet, the intestinal wall may allow some of these undigested proteins to pass through. For many people, their body mistakes these proteins for foreign invaders, prompting an immune response. This immune response will, at a minimum, cause gut irritation and inflammation, which, as explained earlier, can lead to a leaky gut.

Things start to get very troubling when the foreign invaders resemble healthy proteins in the body. In some cases the antibodies will attack healthy cells, such as pancreatic proteins, compromising the pancreas. Moreover, a leaky gut is the gateway to several autoimmune diseases, Type I diabetes, celiac disease, and multiple sclerosis, to name a few. Gluten also affects the functioning of glutaminase, which has a hand in modifying every protein in our body—meaning that it has the potential to affect any organ.

It's important to moderate your consumption of all grains, ensuring the ones you do eat are whole grains, and ideally gluten-free (millet, quinoa, amaranth). No matter what you choose, ensure that it is organically grown and always non-GMO. There are many products available, from pasta to breads, that are now using these grains; and, thanks to the rise of gluten intolerance, they are easier to find. It is also important to keep in mind that just because these products are gluten-free doesn't mean there are no consequences in overindulging. In most cases the gluten has been replaced with refined carbs such as rice starch (rice starch may be gluten free but it is a refined carb) and tapioca starch, which may as well be table sugar.

## ii. Dairy

Dairy is often a hot topic in nutritional circles. Some believe it critical for good bone health and calcium intake, while others believe that it's detrimental to our health and should be avoided. Despite our differences of opinion, we were all raised believing that we should eat according to the four food groups and their associated serving recommendations, with dairy as one of these four food groups. Yet another sad reality is that there were a lot of political motivations for promoting these four food groups—this is a nice way of saying that powerful lobbyists influenced policy. So once again it's incumbent on us to do our own due diligence to help us understand what we should be eating.

Let's dismiss opinion and analyze the facts. Dairy contains lactose (sugars) and milk fats that are often times difficult to for our bodies to digest. Our bodies need lactase to break down lactose, however as we age, our body's production of lactase decreases, by upwards of 90%. Ineffective processing of lactose can create an acidic environment in the body, hospitable for the growth of harmful bacteria.

In order to metabolize milk fats the liver needs to secrete a type of bile high in sulfur. Again, some harmful bacteria thrive in this environment, causing havoc in the gastrointestinal tract, potentially breaking down the mucosal barrier—which is what allows the stomach to contain its acid. Adding to this is the body's subsequent immune response to these poorly digested fats that creates even more damage to this delicate system. Remember that the billions of friendly bacteria in our gut are our first protection against deadly pathogens. Compromising this environment can lead to a host of immune disorders.

The situation doesn't get any better. Dairy contains casein protein. In animal studies, casein protein consumption above the 10% RDA resulted in exponential growth of foci—cancer precursor cells. It has been shown to act as fuel for tumors. (Campbell TC and Dunaif GE. "Dietary protein level and aflatoxin B1—induced preneoplastic hepatic lesions in the rat." *The Journal of Nutrition* 117 (1987): 1298–1302)

Even if you think dairy is good for you, the romanticized images of dairy production are a thing of the past. Cows are part of a manufacturing process where the majority of them are raised in Caged Animal Feed Operations (CAFOs). In these 'factories', cows are often confined to small feedlots where they show severe signs of stress due to social isolation and the inability to move around or lie down.

Conversely, since the 2010 final ruling by the USDA (Jarvis M, *USDA Issues Final Rule on Organic Acceess To Pasture*, February 2010, USDA), USDA Organic certified farms are required to give cows access to pasture. Disappointingly, as of 2008 less than 1% of all farms in the U.S. were managed organically compared to over 4% in Europe (Willer, Helga; Kilcher, Lukas, 2011, *The World of Organic Agriculture. Statistics and Emerging Trends*. Bonn; FiBL, Frick: IFOAM).

Within these CAFOs, in order for the cows to

produce the most milk possible, operators can employ several techniques, involving antibiotics, growth hormones (rBGH in the U.S.), and over-milking. There are obvious complications with such an aggressive push for production. The cows often become sick and develop infections, which then need to be treated with even more chemicals. Despite safeguards, some studies have found several different chemicals in our milk, including highly toxic compounds such as PCDDs (a dioxin) and dioxin-like compounds, along with puss, pathogens and blood from various infections. (A Schecter, J Startin, C Wright, M Kelly, O Päpke, A Lis, M Ball, and J R Olson "Congener-specific levels of dioxins and dibenzofurans in U.S. food and estimated daily dioxin toxic equivalent intake." Environ Health Perspect 102(11) (1994): 962–966,). Hence the need for milk to be pasteurized before packaging. Pasteurization, however, along with killing any bacteria, compromises some of the nutritional value of the milk.

If you really need or want to continue consuming milk it would be best to buy from a certified organic dairy farmer. As another alternative, organic goat or sheep's milk is often better tolerated by people with dairy sensitivities. The best option would be to seek out organic coconut or almond milk.

> ### Ikkuma **INFO**
>
> **Recombinant Bovine Growth Hormone (rBGH):** This growth hormone is a synthetic version of a hormone produced naturally in the cow's pituitary glands. Its main purpose is to increase the cow's milk production. Although rBGH is banned in Canada, the EU and several other countries, it's injected in nearly a third of all cows in the U.S. Once again the U.S. trails the rest of the world in protecting its citizens. Moreover, the milk produced from these cows has elevated levels of the hormone IGF-1. This hormone messes with your pituitary glands, having adverse effects on your metabolic and hormonal balance. In excess, it is also linked to higher rates of many cancers. (Daxenberger A, Breier BH, Sauerwein H. "Increased milk levels of insulin-like growth factor 1 (IGF-1) for the identification of bovine somatotropin (bST) treated cows." *Analyst*. 1998 Dec. 123 (12):2429–35)

### iii. Sugar & Fructose

Let's review some startling facts about sugar:

- Americans consume over 90 pounds of sugar annually, on top of what they consume naturally from fruits and vegetables—this is well over the amount needed to cause metabolic dysfunction (Taubes G. "Is Sugar Toxic?", April 13, 2011, *The New York Times*)

- In the American Heart Association journal *Circulation*, a study following approximately 43,000 men for over 20 years reported that simply consuming one 12-ounce sweetened beverage per day would increase the likelihood of a heart attack by 20%.

These are just two of the hundreds and hundreds of jaw-dropping stats related to sugar consumption in the Western world. Sugar consumption has truly gotten beyond out of control.

Sugar (sucrose) is composed of equal parts glucose and fructose. When sugar is consumed, your pancreas produces insulin to shuttle the sugar where it is needed, namely your muscles and your brain. Your liver then metabolizes the rest, either storing it or producing fatty acids (which are subsequently stored as fat). With excessive sugar consumption, the cells in your body become increasingly insulin resistant due to a myriad of factors, one being fatty acid overload. The pancreas then needs to work harder and harder to produce more and more insulin. Eventually, when insulin resistance reaches critical levels, the stage is set for type II diabetes.

Leptin is another hormone affected by excess sugar consumption. Excessive sugar consumption decreases leptin sensitivity, which, as mentioned earlier, is key for controlling hunger. When leptin sensitivity decreases, the signal to stop eating is weakened, leading to even more overconsumption.

It's a vicious circle that leads to obesity and other related diseases, such as metabolic syndrome. Metabolic syndrome, easily defined, is a combination of risk factors—insulin resistance, elevated cholesterol and high blood pressure (hypertension)—which increase the probability of diseases such as CVD, stroke, and diabetes. It is caused by overall metabolic dysfunction and driven by unhealthy habits, such as excessive sugar/fructose consumption.

### *Ikkuma* **INFO**

**Surprising Sugar in Common Foods:** We need to be very wary of many of the foods we eat, in that they have surprisingly high amounts of sugar. Keep in mind that a safe level of sugar for the average consumer is approximately 25 grams per day. Here are some surprising foods that have sugar comparable to a candy bar:

- Canned Fruit: even fruit needs to be consumed in moderation. Canned fruit is often packed in syrup that is loaded with sugar. Some products contain over 30 grams of sugar.
- Tomato Sauce: this seemingly healthy food packed with

cancer fighting lycopene, often has added sugar. This added sugar, as well as the pasta it's typically eaten with, can create a significant sugar spike.
- Fat-Free Salad Dressing: often time fats are replaced with fillers such as sugars and starches. Fats are not inherently evil. Carbs are a bigger concern for obesity and chronic disease.
- Yogurt: many yogurts have added sugar or artificial sweeteners (which I will discuss shortly). They often contain artificial colors and flavors. Look for unsweetened, or naturally sweetened, organic, full-fat yogurts. As you now know, fat-free is often full of replacement sugars.
- Muffins: even bran muffins almost always contain a large amount of sugar to make them edible. Muffins are essentially pure carbs, packing well over 30 grams of sugar.
- Granola bars: granola is often construed as being very healthy. The sad truth is that most granola bars have sugar as the #1 ingredient. Even the granola itself is a potent carb, in that it eventually gets metabolized into sugar.

One type of sweetener that we need to be very aware of is high fructose corn syrup (HFCS). High fructose corn syrup is found in an incredible percentage of the processed food you'll find at the supermarket. Corn, which is highly subsidized in the U.S., is artificially inexpensive, resulting in corn based sweeteners as the sweeteners of choice for food processors. You'll find this sweetener anywhere companies can stick it, and they find incredible places to stick HFCS. Remember, a lot of companies out there are constantly looking for cheap shit to put in their food. Luckily, high fructose corn syrup is the 'cheap-shit' king, so companies love it.

Every cell in your body uses glucose, with typically about 20% metabolized by your liver; whereas the liver needs to metabolize nearly 100% of the fructose you consume because it alone is equipped to handle it—in a process called fructolysis. Hence, consumed in excess, fructose can overtax the liver, damaging it much like excessive alcohol consumption. This can lead to NAFLD (non-alcoholic fatty liver disease), which, terrifyingly enough, is actually starting to affect children! (Nobili V., Marcellini M., Devito R., et al. "NAFLD in children: A prospective clinical-pathological study and effect of lifestyle advice." July 2006, *Hepatology*)

The key to understanding the dangers of fructose lies in understanding how it affects our bodies, and how the body metabolizes it. It is has been observed that fructose depletes the energy of a cell, preventing it from functioning normally, causing oxidative stress, and inflammation. Fructose is also responsible for creating advanced glycation enzymes (AGEs), which accelerate the aging process.

Some theorize that fructose promotes obesity, not due to the calories, but due to a specific physiological response in body. Fructose activates a key enzyme, fructokinase, which in turn activates another enzyme that promotes fat accumulation in cells. You could liken fructose to a fat storage switch.

The horror story continues. Fructose effectively sabotages your appetite management system, in that it doesn't adequately stimulate insulin production, resulting in a state where the body does not suppress your hunger hormone (ghrelin) but suppresses the satiety hormone (leptin). This suppression double-whammy has a dangerous domino effect, as the increase in appetite will cause a person to eat more, which in turn can lead to insulin resistance, metabolic syndrome, and potentially type 2 diabetes and heart disease. Research has shown metabolic syndrome to be similar to that of hibernating mammals. They have fat storage conditions, with all the same symptoms of metabolic syndrome—fatty liver, increased triglycerides and insulin resistance (much like alcoholism, see Ikkuma Info on next page). Supporting this, studies in rats have also shown that fructose promoted a metabolic syndrome-type condition that did not appear in rats that were fed glucose.

Fructose in its whole food form (ie: an apple vs. apple juice) is less of a shock for the body to deal with. This is because fruit contains other macronutrients, such as fiber, that slow the entry of fructose into the bloodstream. Fructose outside of whole food, such as high fructose corn syrup, is the true culprit.

> ### *Ikkuma* **INFO**
>
> **Toxic Effect of Fructose vs. Alcohol:** Amazingly, fructose and alcohol affect the liver in very similar ways. Since the liver metabolizes nearly 100% of the fructose you consume, it can overload the liver much like excessive alcohol. They have very similar toxic effects, namely visceral fat, fatty liver, metabolic syndrome and insulin resistance. Fructose is also believed to stimulate the pleasure centers of the brain, encouraging people to over-consume, much like a narcotic. Like alcohol, fructose consumption needs to be controlled.

So remember, never believe "a calorie is a calorie". All calories are not made equal. One key difference between consumption of fructose versus glucose, protein, or fats is the hormonal response they ellicit. Even if you consume the same number of calories from each, they will have very different effects on how much fat you accumulate. Remember, with the exception of post-workout or fasting induced glycogen depletion, that nearly 100%

of the fructose you consume gets metabolized by your liver. Fructose is also several times more reactive than glucose in producing advance glycation end products, which is key to accelerating the aging process. Glucose and fructose are very different animals.

### iv. Artificial Sweeteners

If high fructose corn syrup is the 'cheap-shit' king then artifical sweeteners are the 'evil' prince. At least you know what you're getting with high fructose corn syrup—crap (has that sunk in yet?).

Artifical sweeteners, on the other hand, are a much more complex an animal. While believed to help with weight management, they actually induce carb cravings, stimulate your appetite, and promote weight gain (fat storage). The various types of sweeteners—aspartame (eg. Equal), sucralose (eg. Splenda), and acesulfame potassium (eg. Acesulfame-K)—have various claims against them, from causing neurological damage, to having carcinogenic properties and wreaking havoc on gut health. I literally have a hard time keeping my food down if I know it has artificial sweeteners. Read on and maybe you'll feel the same.

Though there are several out there, let's focus our attention toward the two most popular: aspartame and sucralose.

Aspartame has a sullied history that few know about. It took several votes before the FDA somehow approved aspartame fit for use in the early 80s (after originally being approved in the early 70's and appealed). As Dr. Mercola explains in *"Artifical Sweeteners: More Sour Than You Ever Imagined"* (www.mercola.com) aspartame has been linked to several adverse effects such as seizures, nausea, and anxiety attacks. The main components of aspartame are the chemicals phenylalanine, aspartic acid, and methanol, each of which pose a specific danger to humans:

- An abundance of phenylalanine in your brain can cause mood disorders by decreasing serotonin levels.
- Excess aspartic acid can destroy neurons due to allowing excess calcium to penetrate your cells.
- Lastly, the oxidation of methanol inside the body creates toxins, such as formaldehyde, which are toxic and carcinogenic.

Even moderate consumption of aspartame introduces levels of methanol in the body well above the EPA recommended dosage (Mercola Dr. *Aspartame is, by far, the most dangerous substance on the market that is added to foods.* November 2011)

Although both phenylalanine and aspartic acid are found in many proteins (in proper combinations with other amino acids), when they are consumed as isolated amino acids they are no longer inert and become harmful. As reported by the FDA, aspartame is responsible for more reports of adverse reactions than all other food and food additives combined.

Next on the list is sucralose, which was approved by the FDA in 1998. In animal studies, this sweetener has been shown to severely reduce—by upwards of 50%—the amount of good bacteria in the gut and digestive tract, and actually contributes to increases in body weight (Abou-Donia MB, El-Masry EM, et al. "Splenda alters gut microflora and increases intestinal p-glycoprotein and cytochrome p-450 in male rats" *Journal of Toxicology and Environmental Health* Part A 2008: 71(21):1415–29). It's an unnatural sweetner that veils itself as an alternative to sugar, where it should be anything but.

When we consume, empty, artificially sweetened, no-calorie foods, they increase our craving for more carbohydrate-rich foods. Remember that sugars are carbohydrates, and carbohydrates are the body's fuel. We have a hunger for carbohydrates for a reason—energy! Our brains have been hardwired to expect calories when they encounter sweetness, and when this caloric reward does not occur it craves that void to be filled. So while we think that consuming sugar-free sweets helps us lose weight, in actuality they increase our cravings for more full-calorie carbohydrates.

Artifical sweetners are not necessary, and are easy to phase out of your diet. Pay special attention to anything sugar-free because if it's sweet, chances are it has artificial sweetener added. Better alternatives to artificial sweeteners are stevia and pure dextrose.

### v. Alcohol

*"The problem with some people is that when they aren't drunk, they're sober."*
—W.B. YEATS, IRISH POET

*"First you take a drink, then the drink takes a drink, then the drinks takes you."*
—F. SCOTT FITZGERALD, AMERICAN NOVELIST

As I've mentioned, I was a vice-president for an alcohol company. I never try to misrepresent myself. I won't lie. I've been known to have the odd cocktail, and by odd I mean several. I make a lot of Ikkuma Account deposits to indulge now and then. But I do have my limits and know them well, and for the most part, abide by them.

Alcohol's not all bad. In moderation it's known to help increase good (HDL) cholesterol, reduce the formation of blood clots, and potentially help prevent arterial damage caused by bad LDL cholesterol. Because of this, alcohol is said to have positive effects on hypertension and cardiovascular disease.

Alcohol in moderation means a lot of different things to a lot of different people. Doing belly shots after finishing off a 26'er is not moderation. Moderation looks more like a couple of drinks a day for men and one for women. In these quantities you reap the beneficial effects of alcohol, regardless of the alcohol you choose. The difference in recommended quantities lies in the fact that men usually weigh more and typically have more of the enzyme that metabolizes alcohol. Some swear by red wine due to its resveratrol content, but as reported by the Mayo Clinic in their article, *Red wine and resveratrol: Good for your heart?*, you would need to drink over 60 liters of wine to mimic the amounts of resveratrol shown to have beneficial effects in mice studies.

Take note—there are still risk factors to drinking daily, including increased cancer risk. If you continually abuse alcohol, you can seriously compromise your liver, lose water soluble vitamins (specifically B's) and reduce insulin's effectiveness—much like the effect of a very poor diet. This is not a revelation. Alcohol consumption can become habit forming, so in no way am I advocating for people to start drinking to improve their health. Yet, if you do enjoy a drink here and there, it may actually be helping you in the long run.

## vi. Trans Fats (Trans fatty acids)

Manmade trans fats have been around for over 50 years. Remember all those cookies and cakes we grew up with? Chances are they had an unhealthy helping of trans fats. Trans fats are essentially polyunsaturated corn or soy oils, superheated with added hydrogen. They have the resilience of saturated fats, in that they are stable in processed foods over long periods of time, but wreak havoc on the liver in different ways.

As we definitively learned in the 1990's, trans fats are indeed an extremely destructive invention. They have been linked to several debilitating conditions such as cancer and hormonal imbalances. They have also been found to increase LDL cholesterol ("bad") and lower HDL cholesterol ("good"), which increases the risk of heart disease (Mayo Clinic Staff, *Trans Fat Is Double Trouble For Your Heart Health*, Mayo Clinic 2011 May). There are some arguments that trans fats are no worse that saturated fats, however a study conducted in 2004, reported in *Atherosclerosis, Thrombosis and Vascular Biology*, illustrated that trans fats had a more detrimental effect on heart healthy HDL cholesterol when compared to saturated fats.

The government now strictly controls trans fats, including requiring labeling in processed foods, making it easier to eliminate them from your diet. In places like New York City, trans fats are actually banned from restaurants. This is definitely a step in a long overdue right direction.

## We have a choice...

At this point in the book I can't help but reflect on the food processing inventions of the past several decades. It's important that everyone takes the time to reflect on the advent of food processing, and mechanically engineered food products.

Ask yourselves if manufactured food has truly improved the quality of our health. In my opinion, once you start looking at the facts about how these refined, manufactured and processed foods react in your body, and the correlations between them and increased incidences of disease, it just makes sense to cut them out of your diets.

Furthermore, despite being known to cause serious damage to public health, the companies responsible for these pseudo-nutritional foods continue to come across as if they are designing products to improve our health, or reduce its price and increase the availability of quality food, when really, their sole interest lies in financial gain. The food industry, along with government regulators, should be ashamed at what the general public has been exposed to in the past 50 years. We have effectively become experimental rats in financially lucrative laboratory experiments. There was nothing wrong with food choices in the early 1900's. While our ancestors did not have access to the variety of whole foods we have now, nearly everything they ate was grown, not processed.

The answers are simple. The question is: what are you prepared to sacrifice to create the healthy body you want? Are you prepared to go with one less electronic gadget, or spend that extra 15 minutes to prepare a proper meal instead of an instant dinner? These are not choices I can make for you, however I hope you now feel equipped to make better choices for yourself.

Stop bullshitting yourself into thinking that you'll get away with these questionable lifestyle decisions. The Canadian Cancer Society predicts that, on average, the last ten years of our lives will be spent battling disease. Go to your nearest hospital and see if you like the digs. If your going to be sick for ten years, you better get used to it. Better yet, ask some chronic disease sufferers what they think. Stop the cycle now. Make changes.

### **SECTION TWO** PART TWO: FOODS TO 'DRIVE BY'

#### Ikkuma Top *Foods To 'Drive' By* Tweets:

- **Wheat** has undergone several changes over time. It's high in gluten (an issue for many) and often overly processed. **Choose healthier grains.**
- **Milk**, a diet staple for years, is difficult for the body to metabolize and acidic in nature. **Opt for vegetables as great calcium sources.**
- In the U.S., **rBGH**—increases milk production and known to be harmful—is still legal for use in cattle. **Avoid it!** http://huff.to/13P2SRE
- **High fructose corn syrup** is linked to rampant obesity. Nearly 100% of fructose directly hits the liver. **Nuff said.** http://huff.to/17UEjo7
- Many apparently healthy foods have loads of **sugar. Read the label and make smart choices.** Some foods will shock you http://bit.ly/17UEP5y
- To combat fat gain from processed and sugary foods, try **intermittent fasting.** See my Ikkuma Info: Intermittent Fasting.
- **Ditch the artificial sweeteners.** Don't be fooled by their zero calorie claims. They're toxic and induce overeating. http://bit.ly/13ptGsh
- **Alcohol in moderation**—1 to 2 drinks per day—can be beneficial. Binge drinking can be very toxic to your liver and is highly acidic.

- **Avoid trans fats** or any other food with hydrogenated on the label. They tax your heart and lead to weight gain http://mayocl.in/160tPG6

### Bonus Ikkuma *Foods To 'Drive' By* Tweets:

- Avoid foods with health claims. Selling us on fortified foods is just another gimmick to fake nutrition. Real food doesn't need a claim.
- Beware of "natural flavoring". It is often disguising the presence of MSG, which stimulates your brain to eat more http://bit.ly/1224VPW

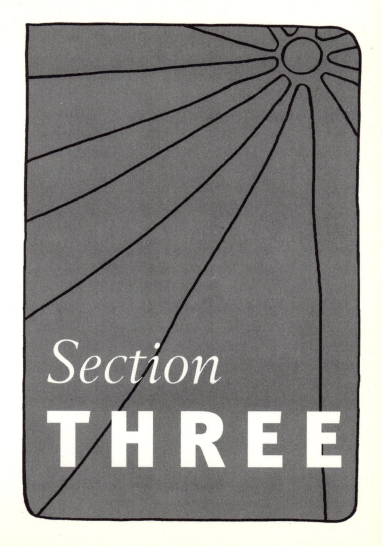

# Toxins...
# The Ugly Truth

*(Ikkuma Translation: 'Get That Tire Out of the Fire!')*

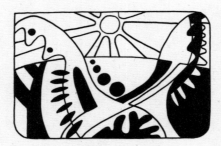

"Learn to live in balance"—"When we open our eyes to the underlying wholeness of life, our actions will shift. Nature will again become our partner in the creation of a conscious healthy world."—S. LeBlanc

*"Our own physical body possesses a wisdom which we who inhabit the body lack. We give it orders which make no sense."*
—HENRY MILLER, AMERICAN AUTHOR

In talking about organics earlier in the book you were sensitized to the ubiquity of toxins, and their far reaching effects on humans and the environment—it effectively began the discussion. This section will continue this discussion and dive into much more detail. The end in mind for this section is for you, the reader, to gain insight on the toxic dangers out there and feel confident that reasonable choices can be made. Let's start by refreshing ourselves with the scope of our toxic overload.

Oh I love the 'toxin lovers' who argue this one. They contend that there is an acceptable limit of toxins. Who cares! Stop rationalizing this crap. I might be able to take a punch in the head and survive, but do I want my business partner to start pummeling me (although in this case he probably would kill me).

Toxins are bad. We've been taught this since our parents showed us the skull and crossbones on the chlorine bottle. So, if you could understand that as a 4 year old, tell me when your head entered your ass and somehow forgot.

The challenge lies in that fact that it's not always as obvious as a skull and crossbones on a bottle. Don't fret because this is your lucky day. I'm going to put a big, virtual skull and crossbones on most things you shouldn't be exposed to.

We know toxins are in the environment. A U.S. EPA report in 2002 stated that over seven billion pounds of over 600 different types of chemicals, were released into the water and air. Seven billion pounds! How does this translate into understanding their effect on humans? Unfortunately, there is no exact method to ascertain what a non-toxic level to humans represents, because we are all physiologically unique and controlled studies are all but impossible. What we do know is that no toxins are better than some toxins. I know this sounds juvenile, but since we know so little about what a safe dose is, to me it seems irrefutable to strive for anything other than zero.

There are examples of toxins' effects everywhere. Some of the most troubling examples are found in common items our children interact with on a daily basis, including toys, shower curtains, and vinyl flooring. The average person would never have thought that these items could be a detriment to our children's health, but studies have shown that the phthalates (man-made chemical) found in these common household items is actually getting into our bloodstream. What effect this then has on our children, and us, is highly debatable, however some experts believe they are affecting reproductive development, and potentially acting as endocrine disruptors (affecting the functioning of our hormones) (Foss K, "Clues to the early puberty mystery," *Health Reporter*, March 2009).

In any event, the evidence is piling up. We are slowly beginning to understand toxins' effects on the human body, both in the short and long term. What will be the next banned substance that we have been treating as benign? Asbestos and BPA have been past culprits.

Before we get into all the various chemicals and sources of these chemicals, let's develop an understanding of how they can effect us. When discussing toxins' overall effects on humans, there are two main categories that adverse chemical exposure fall under: toxic chemical reactions or chemical sensitivities. It is important for people who believe they have been exposed to a chemical to try and distinguish between the two in order to properly determine a course of action.

A *toxic chemical reaction* is an *acute* response after being exposed to a certain chemical. Typically, the symptoms are similar for all exposed and heighten in severity as the chemical exposure increases. On the other hand, someone who has a specific *chemical sensitivity* can become *progressively* more ill even as the exposure levels decrease. The symptoms are often unique and isolated to each case, which is why diagnosing chemical sensitivies can be difficult. Acute reactions to a chemical are possible, but chronic, multiple chemical sensitivities are more likely.

Our bodies need to work overtime to deal with all the chemicals we are now exposed to. Many of these toxins and heavy metals that we are exposed to on a daily basis are fat-soluble, and therefore must be processed by the liver, then eliminated from the body through either the bowel or the kidneys. This process gets sabotaged by increasingly, and commonly, over-burdened livers, which contributes to chemical sensitivities. In this scenario the liver is unable to keep up with the amount of toxins it is required to process, allowing these toxins to build up in the body; particularly in our fat and bones.

The liver, though incredibly important for detoxification, isn't alone in the body's fight to eliminate toxins; it is supported by five other channels of elimination, namely the kidneys, bowel, lymphatic system, lungs and skin. They all work together in an attempt to rid the body of waste. But as I said earlier, we are chemically over-exposed as a society, and these channels often cannot keep up. As Doris Rapp highlights in *Our Toxic World: A Wake Up Call* (Environmental Medical Research Foundation, 2004), symptoms associated with chemical sensitivities often include headaches, sensitivities to smells such as perfume, numbness, and skin irritation. These symptoms can be immediate or can manifest themselves over days, or weeks. For some, exposure can lead to serious brain and nervous system damage, manifesting itself as memory loss or physical and mental debilitation.

Rapp goes on to highlight that in the U.S., upwards of 70 million people are believed to have chemical sensitivities of some kind. Many of these people have reactions to the most benign of sources, such as paint or perfume. Often times individuals who are chemically sensitive have pre-existing conditions such as asthma, or allergies, which can make an individual even more sensitive to toxins, and often worsen their condition. Of those affected, approximately 10 million are so severely affected that they cannot function normally outside of a sterile environment. It is incredible how little awareness there is for such a pervasive issue.

Before we get in depth on typical and common toxic sources, let's quickly highlight some of the main chemicals out there and how they can be avoided:

## Main chemicals we're exposed to

| Chemical: Triphenyltin (herbicides) | | |
| --- | --- | --- |
| Source | Effects | How to Avoid |
| Antifungal paints and fungicides | Permanent adverse effects on one's immune system. | Pay attention to chemical declarations and avoid those products. |

| Chemical: Organichlorides (pesticides) | | |
| --- | --- | --- |
| Still often used on lawns under the chemicals 2,4-D and 2,4,5-T and treated wood | Linked to higher incidences of cancer, such as lymphoma. | Opt for natural fertilizers and question how your deck wood has been treated. |

| Chemical: Organophosphates (pesticides) |||
|---|---|---|
| **Source** | **Effects** | **How to Avoid** |
| May be sprayed in municipal parks and common areas under the chemical malathion | Shown to cause serious nervous system damage. | Question your municipality on how they control pests. Control where your children play. |
| **Chemical: Carbamates** |||
| Clothing and plastics | Not as toxic as some of the previously listed chemicals but may effect several organs. | In the least, ensure clothes are washed before wearing. Organic fabrics are ideal but not yet practical to obtain. |
| **Chemical: Phthalates** |||
| Floor tiles, plastics, shower curtains and various adhesives—in the fumes | Believed to act as serious endocrine (hormonal) disruptors. | This gets tricky. Replace what can be replaced, such as shower curtains. Opt for wooden toys if practical. |
| **Chemical: Solvents** |||
| Common solvents are benzene, toluene, and xylene | Adverse effects can range from cancer to kidney damage. | Ensure there is ample ventilation if you ever need to use solvents. Avoid breathing them in. |

**SECTION THREE:** TOXINS... THE UGLY TRUTH

We're getting closer to understanding the issue, what's out there, and a few specific offenders. Now I feel it important to list the wide range of symptoms you may experience due to chemical sensitivities and heavy metal toxicity, because many of us go years with symptoms, or without being able to identify the root cause.

Here is a list of potential symptoms of chemical sensitivity:

- Fatigue
- Headaches
- Attention deficit
- Muscle aches
- Itchy eyes and runny nose
- Coughing
- Joint pain
- Metallic taste
- Ear, nose or throat infections
- Rashes
- Insomnia
- Gastrointestinal distress
- Unusual behavior

This list is not exhauastive and meant to be directional in nature. Our challenge lies in the fact that many of these symptoms are non-specific, meaning that they can be due to many different things, and are often lived with and accepted. Although this is often the case, some chemical sensitivities or heavy metal toxicities can be tested for, and treated. A visit to a naturopathic doctor is advisable if you suffer from any of these symptoms.

It is important for a person to honestly assess ailments they have, try and find, and then remove the source. It is often not enough to simply remove the source, however, as many toxins are fat-soluble and as such need to be actively removed. Food sensitivities may behave in a similar fashion, in that you can remove the food, but detoxification and healing need to occur in order for your system to rebalance itself. In both cases naturopathic medicine has holistic techniques to help detoxify and rebalance the body.

## I just ate what?!

If you knew the chemicals used to grow your conventional food, you may think twice before chowing down. In fact, the EPA reported that in 2007 approximately 857 million pounds of conventional pesticide was used in the U.S. alone, with about 80% used on cropland. This is nearly three pounds per citizen. Is this truly necessary for us to grow our food? Even with all these chemicals being used, yield loss due to pests continues to challenge farmers. Complicating matters, the over-application of pesticides is giving birth to new superpests, which are becoming stronger and more resilient.

Perhaps coincidentally—though I am highly doubtful that it is—our children are increasingly being diagnosed with autism, allergies, attention deficit, and cancer. These correlations are becoming increasingly difficult to accept when we are finding babies that are being born with measurable levels of various chemicals in their blood, such as DDT, DDE, and PCBs. They are literally being born toxic. And these chemicals are not shown to be inert either; as correlations have been made between weight gain and exposure to these chemicals, potentially due to these chemicals acting as endocrine (hormone) disruptors. (Valvi D, Mendez M, et al. "Prenatal Concentrations of Polychlorinated Biphenyls DDE, DDT and Overweight Children: A Prospective Birth Cohort Study." *Environmental Health Perspectives*, October 2011).

Toxic exposure starts at childbirth, with chemicals tending to build up in our systems over the years, which are then deposited and stored in our fat tissue. A 1996 EPA report found that adults over the age of 45 had over 5 times the levels of chemical pesticides in their fat stores, compared to children under the age of 14 (Lordo R, Dinh K, et al. "Semivolatile Organic Compounds in Adipose Tissue: Estimated averages for the US Population and Selected Subpopulations" *American Journal of Public Health*, 1996 Sep; 86(9):1253–9.

Things are definitely not improving. As I've harped on repeatedly, today we're exposed to massive amounts of pesticides and herbicides in and on our food, with chemicals once deemed to be safe, such as BPA (often a component in old baby bottles), now outlawed in certain countries. What other apparently safe chemicals on the market today will be deemed dangerous in the future?

There are several sources of chemicals, including our food, that we need to be aware of. The Environmental Working Group (www.ewg.com)—a leading American environmental health research and advocacy organization—has done a great job outlining the most contaminated conventionally grown foods and those with the least pesticide contamination, in the U.S., as outlined in the Table below.

## The "Dirty Dozen" & the "Clean Fifteen"

| "The Dirty Dozen" | "The Clean Fifteen" |
|---|---|
| Apples | Asparagus |
| Bell Peppers | Avocado |
| Blueberries (Domestic) | Cabbage |
| Celery | Cantaloupe (Domestic) |

| Cucumbers | Corn |
| --- | --- |
| Grapes | Eggplant |
| Lettuce | Grapefruit |
| Nectarines (imported) | Kiwi |
| Peaches | Mangoes |
| Potatoes | Mushrooms |
| Spinach | Onions |
| Strawberries | Pineapples |
| | Sweet Peas |
| | Sweet Potatoes |
| | Watermelon |

## Fluoride

I'd like to change gears a little and focus on one chemical that we regularly ingest, under the guise of "safe for consumption". Many of us still use fluorinated toothpaste, drink fluorinated water and grew up with fluoride treatments. Remember when the dentist used to soak your teeth in fluoride for 10 minutes or so? It was sold to the public on the premise that it strengthened your enamel, yet added fluoride is not essential for human health, dental or otherwise.

Fluoride, like many other fat soluble toxins, accumulates in our tissues. Although much of the fluoride you ingest exits your body, the vast majority of what remains is absorbed and accumulates in tissues such as teeth, bones and even blood vessels. There are nutrients that bind to fluoride, working to reduce its accumulative effects, however no amount of fluoride is a good thing.

Besides being commonly known as a carcinogen, fluoride has been associated with compromising your immune system, brain damage, and accelerated aging. Educate yourself on what is in your water and choose fluoride free toothpaste. Why take unnecessary risks when you don't need to?

> ### *Ikkuma* **INFO**
>
> **Mercury:** up to 50% of dentists in the U.S. still use dental amalgam for fillings, which hovers at around 50% mercury content. Mercury is a well-known vaporous neurotoxin that builds up in fatty tissue, especially the brain. It can seriously harm your kidneys and create a host of neurological issues. It is still used by dentists because it's quick and easy. Amalgams are also one of the biggest sources of mercury in the environment, where even minute amounts can contaminate water tables. Don't expose your children to this true threat.

**SECTION THREE:** TOXINS... THE UGLY TRUTH

## What you don't eat can still hurt you

There are countless toxins we are exposed to that we do not ingest, at least not knowingly. Unbeknownst to many out there, toxins creep into our bloodstream via our biggest organ, the skin. Think of the nicotine patch. It's applied on the skin with the medication then absorbed into your bloodstream to have a desired effect. The technical term for this is transdermal absorption. That's why knowing what goes on your skin is so critical, yet so often underestimated.

I think this is another area where we try to convince ourselves that spending the extra money for organic, or even simple natural products, isn't worth it. I know that feeling when you save $3 on your sunscreen and are ecstatic that your saving the few bucks. In the end what's $3 when, for the next two months, that crap will smother your body, and your child's body, every time you get sun. Shortly, I'll be digging a little deeper into the potential dangers lurking in your sunscreen.

Look, not everything that touches your skin gets absorbed but a heck of a lot does. When you go cheap on what goes in or on your body, the only person your cheating is yourself. You know this. And trust me, there are measurable consequences.

Toxins you apply topically can be contained in anything from make-up to soaps or skin lotions. I also lump electromagnetic fields from cell phones in this category. We cannot possibly talk about all the dangers out there but the table below lists some of the most common sources and what to look for to protect yourself.

## Common sources of chemicals in your daily life

| Product: Shampoo | | | |
|---|---|---|---|
| **Average number of chemicals** | **Most Dangerous** | **Associated Issues** | **How to Avoid** |
| >10 | Sodium lauryl sulphate, tetra sodium, propylene glycol | Irritation, possible eye damage | Read the label and look for organic or at least find natural sources, while avoiding these chemicals. |
| **Product: Eye Shadow** | | | |
| >25 | Polyethylene terephthalate | Organ damage, links to cancer, hormonal disruption | There are many natural or organic options for make-up and cosmetics. Read the label. |

**SECTION THREE:** TOXINS... THE UGLY TRUTH

| Product: Lipstick | | | |
|---|---|---|---|
| **Average number of chemicals** | **Most Dangerous** | **Associated Issues** | **How to Avoid** |
| >30 | Polymenthyl methacrylate | Allergies, links to cancer | There are many natural or organic options for make-up and cosmetics. Read the label. |
| **Product: Fake Tanner** | | | |
| >20 | Various parabens | Irritation, hormonal disruption | Get some sun instead. |
| **Product: Perfume** | | | |
| >200 | Benzaldehyde | Links to kidney damage, irritation to mouth and throat | Essential oils are chemical free. Many excellent perfumes offer these options. |
| **Product: Hairspray** | | | |
| >10 | Octinoxate, isophthalates | Hormonal disruption, allergies, irritation to throat & eyes | Read the label and avoid. The toxins become airborne and you breathe them in directly. |

| Product: Foundation | | | |
| --- | --- | --- | --- |
| Average number of chemicals | Most Dangerous | Associated Issues | How to Avoid |
| >20 | Polymenthyl methacrylate | Allergies, links to cancer | There are many natural or organic options for make-up and cosmetics. Read the label. |
| Product: Body Lotion | | | |
| >30 | Various parabens | Irritation, hormonal disruption | There are a plethora of organic options out there. |

### i. Sunscreens

I purposely have not included sunscreens in the previous table. I wanted to specifically highlight sunscreens—the product that we have been sold on as safe and obligatory for any sun exposure. This campaign to justify sunscreen's obligtory use is probably one of the most lucrative fear campaigns ever conducted… and this one vilified the sun.

Since sunscreens are so ubiquitous, I think it's worth highlighting some of the dangers. Writer D.H. Lawrence aptly sums up our relationship with the sun, "If we think about it, we find that our life consists in a relation with all things; stone, earth, trees, flowers, water, insects, fishes, birds, creatures, sun, rainbow, children, women, other men. But his greatest and final relation is with the sun." Yet sadly, over time, we have grown to fear the sun. I wholeheartedly disagree with the demonization of what gives us life. My greatest fear is not the sun but the lotions we put on our bodies to seemingly protect us. Sunscreens may be one of the most underestimated topically applied toxins we subject our bodies to on a regular basis.

The Environmental Working Group's *2012 Sunscreen Guide* requires the following to make it on its "safe list":

- Contains no oxybenzone or retinyl palmitate (form of vitamin A)
- A maximum spf of 50 (anything stronger is throwing money away)
- Full spectrum protection, i.e. UVA and UVB

Astonishingly, as reported in the guide, only 25% of tested sunscreens are considered free of harmful chemicals and effective at protecting your skin. Remember, many chemicals you put on your skin can find their way into your bloodstream.

So, ironically, many sunscreens may be increasing

our risk of skin cancer and possibly promote the spread of cancer due to their harmful ingredients, namely oxybenzone, retinyl palmitate and various parabens. Let's take a look at these main offenders and claims against them.

Due to its ability to absorb UV rays, oxybenzone is found in approximately half of the sunscreens sold. Some believe it is linked to hormonal disruption and cell damage, potentially leading to cancer. Despite these claims, the FDA still considers it safe and approved for everybody over the age of 6 months.

Retinyl palmitate has been featured in a recent CNN report stating that, "Government funded studies have found that this particular type of vitamin A may increase the risk of skin cancer when used on sun-exposed skin." Moreover, significant amounts of this chemical are readily absorbed through the skin, amplifying the risk. (Dellorto D. *Avoid sunscreens with potentially harmful ingredients, group warns*, May 2012 CNN)

Let's wrap up the discussion by looking at one of the most common ingredients we are exposed to, not only in sunscreens, but in all lotions—parabens. They are chemicals with estrogen-like properties, often referred to as xenoestrogens. Take note that excessive exposure over time of seemingly innocuous estrogen has been linked to increased risk of breast cancer. Wait, there's more. The EPA has linked methyl parabens to hormonal and neurological disruption as well as various cancers. Despite all this we find parabens in many common skin lotions.

On top of reading ingredient labels and making better choices, organic being one of them, when looking for effective sunscreens you should always ensure that they are broad spectrum. This ensures that you are protected against both UVB rays (responsible for sunburns), and UVA rays (can lead to skin damage and aging). Regarding SPF, the range you should be looking at is between 15 and 50 SPF.

### *Ikkuma* **INFO**

**UVA vs. UVB Rays:** UVA rays have a greater wavelength than UVB rays, allowing them to pass through the atmosphere much more effectively. Later in the day our atmosphere actually reflects most UVB rays, while letting UVA rays pass—similar to winter months in the northern hemisphere at any time of day. The bad news is that the rays we want to get are the vitamin D inducing UVBs. UVA rays are most associated with skin damage and cancer. So, get your sun in the middle of the day in moderation and make sure you don't burn.

Throughout *Ikkuma: Evolution of Vitality* all roads lead to caution and logic. Your children may be at risk of long-term ailments due to the products they are exposed to; and all this happens under the claim that these products provide necessary protection. Bottom line, if you are buying suntan lotion, look for organic alternatives that use zinc and/or titanium as the active ingredients to protect your skin. There are many great products out there. The Environmental Working Group has a great Sunscreen Guide where they rank sunscreens in terms of safety.

When getting sun, it is always a good idea to err on the side of caution. I often suggest simply starting out with 15 minutes of sun, and, as tolerance increases, you can try to extend this length of time. Remember that the sun is a good thing! Amongst many other benefits, controlled exposure to the sun is a very rich source of vitamin D, whose benefits include, but are not limited to, the following:

- Protects against cancer
- A key ingredient for a healthy heart
- Helps maintain ideal blood pressure
- Supports your immune system

**SECTION THREE:** TOXINS... THE UGLY TRUTH

The sun is not our enemy. It is necessary for all living things and, when respected, is key to long lasting health.

## ii. Household products

We have a slew of chemicals in our homes at any given time. If you take a look at the ingredients in your laundry detergent or air fresheners you will get a taste of the dozens of chemicals you are potentially being exposed to daily. It is literally not even feasible to list them all. But again, since the effects aren't immediately felt, you think you can get away with cheap, synthetic products.

We have no excuses. In this day and age we have access to more natural and organic choices. It could be as simple as finding a more environmentally friendly laundry detergent, or using essential oils to freshen up your house instead of chemical air fresheners (easily found at health food stores). Essential oils are void of synthetic chemicals, making them a better choice for freshening up your house or apartment.

As I touched on earlier, even our clothes can contain toxins. One example, nonylphenol ethoxylate (NPE), is found in many fabrics and detergents sold in the U.S., yet it has been banned in Canada, Europe and several other countries. When introduced in the environment, NPE breaks down into a chemical called nonylphenol.

Once it makes its way into the water it can build up in fish and wildlife. NPEs are a type of xenoestrogen, that is, when NPEs are ingested the organism responds to it much like it responds to estrogen. This is highly toxic and seriously affects the development of the organism. Beyond these hormone disrupting properties, chemicals like NPE may have other wide ranging side effects for the greater human population. (EPA, *Nonylphenol and Nonylphenol Ethoxylates Action Plan Summary*). Admittedly this is difficut to manage but we should be pushing our governments to be more vigilant and grant us more sustainable options.

### iii. Cell Phones

Cell phones represent one of the most disruptive technologies in human history. Now with the advent of smart phones, their impact on our daily lives continues to reach far and beyond what we could have imagined even 10 years ago. Although cell phones have possibly improved our quality of life, the jury is still out on the potential damage that they can have on our health.

Although you may not yet be convinced that cell phones are potentially dangerous, I'm sure many of you have heard reports that the radiation or electromagnetic fields (EMF) they emit is cause for concern.

These potential dangers have caught the attention of the World Health Organization (WHO), who issued a report claiming that cell phones may be carcinogenic (rated as a Class B Carcinogen) due to their radio frequency electromagnetic fields (EMF). (*WHO/IARC Classifies Radiofrequency Electromagnetic Fields as Possibly Carcinogenic to Humans*, May 2011 Electromagnetichealth.org)

In reality, the actual power of a cell phone is quite weak, but even when you are not on a call it emits very erratic radiation, which can potentially interfere with DNA function. We know that our organs are sensitive to radiation and electro-magnetic fields. Unfortunately, since cell phones are still relatively new, we don't know the long-term effects of prolonged cell phone use. There are, however, several studies out there that link cell phone use to increased cancer rates and tumors, especially for women and children. (Hardell, Lennart; Carlberg, Michael; Söderqvist, Fredrik; Mild, Kjell Hansson; Morgan, L. Lloyd (2007). "Long-term use of cellular phones and brain tumors: Increased risk associated with use for ≥10 years". *Occupational and Environmental Medicine 64* (9): 626–32).

Other studies have shown that EMF radiation compromises cell membranes, allowing heavy metals to build up in our system. Heavy metals—such as mercury—are known to negatively impact neurological function, especially in children.

Similar to the discussion regarding GMOs, why not err on the side of caution? I'm not saying ditch the cell phone but there ways you can lower your risk:

- Avoid carrying your cell phone on your body (within 6 inches is most dangerous) and try to turn it off
- Use a headset for phone calls
- Heavily restrict your children from talking extensively on cell phones (I know that this is nearly impossible… just saying!)
- Use a landline when possible (if you actually have access to one)

Now that I've effectively inundated you with about all the toxin-talk you can handle, I'd like to leave you with a few last comments. I may seem like I am exhausting the argument to be wary of toxin exposure in our lives, however it is important to become aware that the disturbing health trends seem to coincide with our dependency on chemicals in our daily lives. For instance, alarmingly, over 1 in 88 children in the U.S. are diagnosed with autism spectrum disorder (ASD), with this rate having risen over 75% in the past five years. Many believe that it stems from the increased toxic exposure that kids are now subject to on a daily basis, while others have cited vaccines as the big culprit. Either way it is a disturbing trend that needs to be better understood.

When it comes to our health and the health of our children, there shouldn't be an acceptable level of risk. It is important to avoid exposure to toxins as much as possible. Eating organic, eliminating toxins from the homes, reducing electro-magnetic fields—such as cell phones, especially in the bedroom, and being concerned with what you put on your skin will minimize the risk.

## Time to detox

The average American will need to detoxify their bodies of hundreds of chemicals they are exposed to daily. Our poor liver is the super organ that takes the brunt of the pain when dealing with all these adulterants. Let's briefly look at how the body deals with this barrage of toxins.

The first phase of detoxification is hepatic (detoxification occurring in the liver). In this phase a number of nutrients are needed to support the liver's ability to detoxify. Through a series of reactions in the liver, supported by nutrients such as B vitamins, toxins get converted into a form suitable for excretion. Once the liver performs its magic, these toxins either travel to the gall bladder where bile taxis it to our colon to be eliminated, or they travel to the kidneys and are excreted via the bladder. If these pathways get clogged, the toxins are either stored inside the body or eliminated through the skin.

With the constant barrage of chemicals in our normal daily lives, we need to ensure that we consume large amounts of healthy foods to obtain the nutrients needed for detoxification; which will help ensure we do not clog the pathways for detoxification. Moreover, avoiding late night meals will allow the liver to finish processing food shortly after midnight, giving it time to recuperate for a busy day ahead.

The toxins that do not get eliminated from the body are stored in fat and tissue. As you burn fat, these toxins get released back into the blood stream. This sets the stage for requiring even more B vitamins and amino acids to deal with the toxic overload. Although this is technically possible, once a toxin penetrates fat and tissue it is very difficult to naturally detoxify. It is important that this be treated on an individualized basis, since we all have varying levels of toxic stress.

Depending on the types of toxins and levels in the body, serious health consequences may result, such as various cancers and neurological disorders. It would be advisable to seek out a naturopathic doctor for rigorous detoxification.

In order to assess your toxin or heavy metal levels, you can simply ask for a chemical screen of your blood and urine through a regulated health professional. If you are found to have elevated levels of toxins or heavy metals in your system, again, seek professional help to detoxify, as naturopathic medicine offers a trusted, individualized approach to removing toxins from the system.

If you are going to try a gentle detox, and depending on the severity of your toxic levels, a great reference for do-it-yourself detoxifying is the book *Natural Detoxification: A Practical Encyclopedia: The Complete Guide to Clearing Your Body of Toxins, 2000* written by Jacqueline Krohn and Frances Taylor (Hartley & Marks 2000).

## *Ikkuma* INFO

**Daily morning cleanse:** Here is what I consider a great daily routine for mild detoxification of the liver.

In the morning, before eating breakfast, immediately take ½ ounce of fresh lemon and drink it with 16 ounces of water. The benefits are unbelievable for something so simple:

- Helps flush out the organs, especially the liver, and kick-starts your metabolism
- Improves your alkaline/acid profile, that is, it promotes alkalinity
- Helps to purge toxins from the body first thing in the morning, which is great for everything including your skin
- Stimulates the birth of new blood and muscle cells
- Helps cleanse the colon, allowing for better nutrient absorption
- Supports your lymphatic system, helping to fight infection

Following this mini- water & lemon cleanse, drink another glass of water, and wait approximately 30 minutes before eating a healthy breakfast. This will give your body enough time to prepare itself to tackle some real food.

## The marvels of modern medicine?

*"Always laugh when you can. It is cheap medicine."*
—Lord Byron, English romantic poet

I've truly attempted to keep my arguments balanced throughout the book. I support holistic—looking at health from all angles—living, but that is simply because all roads lead to this more sustainable and healthy way to live. Despite holistic living being the path to a healthy lifestyle, the conventional health industry is huge, and pharmaceuticals, being a big part of this industry, cannot be ignored.

When I say conventional health 'industry' we really need to absorb what this implies. We're dealing with an industry, not unlike the automotive industry. This industry is judged by the same metrics as any other industry. Do you think that a pharma CEO is more concerned with how many patients' lives were improved by their drugs or how their profits are trending in the existing quarter? I can't speak for every CEO but I would bet that the next board meeting centers around profit projections.

Look, I have come from industry and am not trying to vilify it. What I'm attempting to do is help you realize that, even in the conventional health industry, we are dealing with corporations. And as such, they have a duty to their shareholders to make them as much money as possible. In doing so, there may be times when decisions need to be made in favor of the shareholders, to the detriment of the average main street citizen. Only you can be responsible for your health. Not your doctor and surely not a pharmaceutical company.

### i. Pharmaceuticals

Pharmaceutical drugs are typically designed to treat

people's symptoms, rather than focusing on correcting the root cause of the problem. Judging by your average commercial, however, who the hell would know what any drug is supposed to do? These commercials would have you believe that every time you take a drug, regardless of the symptom, you get teleported to some picturesque field, where the flowers are in bloom and children are frolicking in the lilies. I find that a little misleading, to say the least, because if you've just taken a pill to give you an erection, the last place you want to be is in a field… or is it?

Drugs are also typically very expensive, and involve a wide range of potentially adverse reactions. Just pay attention to the speed talker at the end of a drug commercial.

To protect their industry and get favorable legislation for their drugs, big pharma spends tens of millions of dollars lobbying federal governments. In the U.S., pharmaceutical lobbyists outnumber congressman by approximately two to one (this obviously changes year over year). This 'lobbying' has many outcomes, from suppressing alternative medicine to gaining favorable rulings on potential legislation.

One favorable ruling for the pharmaceutical industry occurred in the 1990's, when direct to consumer drug advertising was allowed; since then the number of chronic drug users has ballooned. The Associated Press reported that in 2007 25% of U.S. children took medication on a regular basis for 'chronic' conditions. We are now being sold on the fact that we need drugs for prevention of chronic illness and that the drugs you used to take occasionally, need to be taken daily. Common medications include ADHD pills, anti-depressants, statins, and hormone replacement medications.

Aspirin is a classic example of an over-used drug. It has been touted to lower the risk of a recurrence of cardiovascular events in patients. It is for this reason that many doctors recommend taking it daily. There are now several findings showing that aspirin does not improve a patient's chance of living longer. In fact, some argue that, because it thins the blood, it actually conceals greater issues until it is too late—the result being a major cardiac event, instead of a gradual onset of symptoms. The side effects of aspirin are well documented, warning mainly of damage to the intestinal tract. Instead of taking aspirin, you can follow the guidelines throughout this book on how to develop a healthy heart naturally. We need to question why pharmaceuticals have now become a normal way of life.

Exacerbating an already dire situation, the FDA is becoming less capable, and potentially lacks the will, to deal with the power of big pharma. As Dr. David Graham, famous whistleblower of the Merck Vioxx scandal—a recall of all Vioxx due to reports of cardiovascular events associated with the drug—stated in 2005, "As currently configured, the FDA is not able to adequately protect the American public. It is more interested in protecting the interests of industry. It views industry as its client, and the client is someone whose interest you represent." (*The FDA Exposed: An Interview With Dr. David Graham, the Vioxx Whistleblower,* August 30, 2005 by: Manette Loudon, Natural News).

Again, I'm not demonizing all Western medicine. I would just lean towards skepticism if you are counting on pharmaceutical companies to look out for your best interests. It is prudent to understand how the drugs you are taking work and their related side effects.

With all that said, treating the root of your specific complaint or illness, instead of the symptom, is much more productive. We are becoming a society dependent on drugs for survival. We are becoming a chronically medicated generation. Western medicine should only be relied on for crisis management. Naturopathic doctors and homeopaths offer much safer alternatives. But always remember that the key to everything is nurturing your body naturally with the proper fuel it needs to thrive.

## ii. Vaccines

I've had more than one heated disagreement with friends regarding vaccines. It's not lost on me that we would be in a much worse position if we didn't have some key vaccines, but I am not convinced our children necessarily require the barrage of vaccines they are faced with today. Since the advent of the smallpox vaccine in 1796, scientists have literally developed hundreds of vaccines.

The general understanding of how vaccines work is as follows: your body's immune system recognizes the vaccine as a foreign invader and, with the help of adjuvants (chemicals added to the vaccine to prompt an immune response), destroys these invaders. In doing so, an immunity to this type of invader is now developed. If ever the virus were to again enter the body, the body would immediately deal with the invader before it picked up any steam. This is obviously oversimplified but you get the picture.

Despite the necessity of certain vaccines, have we now taken the use of vaccines too far? Do we really need a flu vaccine? My generation didn't rely on flu vaccines. We fought whatever bug it was and our immune system adjusted to protect against that virus in the future. Moreover, often times, by the time you get the vaccine—along with its common side effects—for that specific strain, it is already to late. Tragically, society is becoming so dependent on vaccines that we may be creating a generation with compromised, weakened, and unseasoned immune systems. I might sound alarmist, but getting a vaccine just because it's available is not the answer either.

An area of controversy regarding vaccines is the growing speculation that vaccines have been causing cases of autism—though the scientific community does not yet seem to be convinced. There is a case, however, where the Italian Health Ministry concluded that the MMR (measles mumps rubella) vaccine was the cause of a child's autism (Bignell P, "Italian court reignites MMR vaccine debate after award over child with autism" June 2012 *The Independent*). Again, this is an isolated case, which was argued against by several health experts in Britain and other countries.

My advice would be to stick only to what is necessary. Just because a vaccine is available doesn't mean you should take it. Focus on a healthy diet and nurturing your gut flora—the core of your immune system.

### iii. Mammograms and CT Scans

Along with the aggressive evolution in medications, we have seen simlar advances in forms of treatment, such as CT scans and mammograms. These routinely prescribed treatments are, in some cases, doing more harm than good. This represents yet another abuse of medical technology—driven by fear—to increase profits.

Focusing first on mammograms, recent research has shown that they are directly linked to increased risk of breast cancer. I'm not at all suggesting that women avoid mammograms but they should understand that this routine exam is not without its dangers. Women should question their practitioner regarding the frequency and necessity of mammograms.

Most of us are not aware that a mammogram can expose a woman's breast to nearly 1000 times the radiation of a chest x-ray. Unbelievably, according to Dr. Epstein and Dr. Bertell, if pre-menopausal women follow a typical mammogram screening protocol they would be exposed to 5 rads of radiation; this is comparable to the radiation people experienced within one mile of Hiroshima and Nagasaki! (Bertell Dr, Epstein Dr., "The Dangers and Unreliability of Mammography: Breast Examination As A Safe Effective and Practical Alternative," *2001 International Journal of Health Services*). Knowing this, it is not surprising that there have been many studies showing clear correlations between regular mammograms and breast cancer.

There are alternative breast cancer detection methods out there. Ask your doctor about Digital Infrared Imaging. This method of testing can detect changes in breast tissue behavior and does not contain any radiation.

Another common diagnostic tool that involves significant radiation is the CT scan. Although they can be instrumental in diagnosing head injuries and cancer, CT scans too have associated dangers. It has been shown that kids have triple the risk of developing brain cancer after just a few CT scans (Pearce Dr, Salotti J, et al. "Radiation exposure from CT scans in childhood and subsequent risk of leukemia and brain tumors: a retrospective cohort study" August 2012, *The Lancet*, Volume 380, Issue 9840, Pages 499–505, 4 August 2012). Predictably the rate of these treatments being prescribe is skyrocketing. As reported by *CNN Health* (April, 2011), as of 2008 CT Scans have seen a "five fold increase in 14 years".

If CT scans are prescribed:

- ensure that they are necessary
- see if an ultrasound or MRI would be a potential substitute
- request the lowest level of radiation possible

## Individualized Medicine

*"What is food to one, is to others bitter poison."*
　　—LUCRETIUS, ROMAN POET

If I've successfully disuaded you from a future of guzzling down pills, you may be asking yourself, what are the alternatives? Well, you need to attack your health holistically. To achieve and maintain the highest level of health and wellness; diet, supplements, and therapeutic treatment should be individualized.

Everyone is unique genetically, physiologically, biochemically and constitutionally. Whether for health maintenance or disease treatment, it is imperative that an individual's needs are assessed.

Naturopathic medicine applies this philosophy in its practice, using time honored forms of assessment such as Traditional Chinese Medicine (TCM) and homeopathy. Although I will not be digging into it in detail, Ayurvedic medicine is another age old method that incorporates different techniques to ensure the body is in a state of balance.

In TCM the individual's constitution is extremely important in choosing the treatment for illness and imbalance. Tongue and pulse diagnoses are used to assess the health and function of the organs, fluids and the blood of the patient. Based on the findings, the appropriate treatment is chosen, which typically includes a combination of herbs, acupuncture, and food. In TCM, food is viewed as medicine. Conversely, conventional Western medicine typically takes a one-size fits all approach to assessment and treatment, relying too heavily on prescription medication.

Let's use blood pressure to illustrate these differences in philosophy. In North America, conventional treatment would involve following a specific drug protocol in order to reduce blood pressure. If one drug doesn't get the blood pressure to the desired level, they try another, and so on. Assessment and treatment is most commonly based on a standard protocol, and not on the specific needs of the individual. With TCM, five people may all come in with a similar stage of high blood pressure, but they would likely be treated differently, based on their constitution and diagnosis. Rather than focus on the disease itself, treatment would aim at balancing the individual, and addressing the unique origin of the condition.

The second of the more progressive or holistic forms of health assessments I would like to touch on is homeopathy. Homeopathy is one of the most widely used forms of medicine worldwide. It is inexpensive, safe, and effective. The validity and effectiveness of this practice is supported by a massive study conducted in 2011 by the Swiss government on complementary forms of medicine, which included homeopathy.

Homeopathy operates according to the philosophy that "Like Cures Like". It matches the individual's constitution or illness "picture" with a homeopathic substance that will create a similar "picture" in a healthy individual. This is believed to address the imbalance that leads to disease on its highest level, leading to a cure. It is a philosophy difficult for many North Americans to understand, as it is very different from our conventional medical philosophy—coined by the founder of homeopathy, Samuel Hanneman, as the allopathic model.

Now that we have established that food is medicine, let's analyze a few individualized tools used to design one's optimal eating regimen, namely metabolic, blood, and nutritional typing. They represent three methods that may be considered when designing a diet or a program to address the individual's specific needs. Remember that when we look at individual diets and programs for health maintenance, as well as for illness treatment, many factors must be considered in order for the program to have optimal benefit. Factors such as current state of health, nutritional deficiencies, risk factors for disease, family history, personal health history, food sensitivities, genetics and constitution all need to be considered.

Let's delve into metabolic typing a little more closely. Introduced by orthodontist William Donald Kelley, metabolic typing involves catering your nutritional needs to your unique metabolism. Merriam-Webster defines metabolism as "the chemical changes in living cells by which energy is provided for vital processes and activities and new material is assimilated." Kelley leveraged his understanding of diverse types of metabolism to develop the 'Kelley' cancer therapy, which proposed that proper foods for an individual could help combat the deadly disease.

As seen in other forms of individualized nutritional protocols, such as blood or nutritional typing, metabolic typing is premised on the fact that we all have a different make-up or constitution. As such we respond differently to nutritional inputs. In effect:

- we are as unique on the inside as we are on the outside;
- this inherited uniqueness affects physiological systems, structures, and metabolism of cells; these differences imply that we may have individualized nutritional needs

You could liken this to the several different makes of cars. While they all look different on the outside, what we don't see are the infinite mechanical differences on the inside as well. Some run better using regular unleaded gas, while others run better with premium unleaded gasoline. Think of metabolic typing the same way. Some people run better on a high carb regimen, some on a high (meat) protein regimen, and some need a mix. We're all different.

Okay, so now what? We have age old methods of assessing our imbalances and a variety of methods to develop individualized nutritional plans. Why haven't we learned from all this readily available knowledge? Unfortunately, with the help of gratuitous corporate and pharmaceutical profiteering, we have become a society dependent on medication to maintain a symptom-free life; which is very different from a healthy life. If you need to be kept alive by statins (cholesterol lowering medication), or pills to maintain normal blood pressure, then there is something fundamentally wrong. Allopathic medicine is defined by this premise—the premise that we should be treating the symptoms of a condition, not the underlying cause. There is much more money to be made in keeping someone alive on drugs than curing the underlying biochemical imbalances which make up the roots of chronic disease.

A holistic approach to health deals with the root of the illness by correcting the hormonal, nervous, and energy production systems, so that biochemical imbalances (ie: disease) cannot thrive. This approach to health helps ensure that you:

- Effectively treat the root of and prevent chronic illnesses
- Sustain health by dealing with your imbalances
- Treat any condition holistically; treat the body, not the symptom
- Allow your body to perform what it was designed to do—heal itself

Stop the cycle. Avoid toxins as much as humanly possible. Wean yourself off chronic medication by arming your body with the nutrients it needs. And for god's sake, stop treating organic and natural options as discretionary expenses. They're not. Stop looking at the cost for quality goods and make sacrifices in areas of your life that aren't life threatening. Because, believe you me, toxins in every form are life threatening. You know this, so why am I even talking.

### Ikkuma Top *Toxins... The Ugly Truth* Tweets:

- **Be aware of common toxins**, such as solvents, paints and lawn fertilizers.
- If you choose to eat conventional foods, **be aware of the biggest pesticide offenders** in the produce aisle http://bit.ly/10srL15
- **Lose the fluoride toothpaste.** Fluoride is a known

**SECTION THREE:** TOXINS... THE UGLY TRUTH 251

carcinogen. Many cities are banning it from their drinking water.
- In North America mercury is still often used for dental fillings. **Mercury can seriously harm** your kidneys and brain. **Choose safer methods**.
- **Our skin is our biggest organ. Protect it!** Several skincare products, like soaps and lotions, contain known toxins.
- Many **sunscreens contain harmful oxybenzone and parabens. Opt for organic alternatives.** http://bit.ly/ZT9lY5
- **Sun in moderation without sunscreen** is healthy. Shorter wavelength UVB—vitamin D inducing—rays are at their peak at midday.
- The World Health Organization deems the electromagnetic fields associated with **cell phones possibly carcinogenic. Use a bluetooth device.**
- **Choose natural laundry detergents** and fabric softeners. Most household products have several chemicals that we may breath in and absorb.
- The liver is exposed to 100s of chemicals daily. **Eat nutrient rich foods to support detoxification.** Try lemon in water for a morning flush.
- **Vaccines** have been a medical marvel, however they can have adverse effects. **Scrutinize which ones you choose.** Do you really need a flu shot?

- **CT scans** deliver high levels of radiation. Although necessary for serious head trauma, they **should be a last resort.** http://bit.ly/11wQk47
- **Mammography** has been linked to increased incidences of breast cancer. **Opt for alternative screening methods** or reduce mammogram frequency.

## Bonus Ikkuma *Toxins... The Ugly Truth* Tweets:

- **Don't put plastic in the microwave.** Placing plastics in the microwave potentially accelerates its leaching into food and beverages.
- **Avoid xenoestrogens.** These chemicals are notorious for disrupting your hormones. Find them in plastic bottles, pesticides, and PVC curtains.
- **Use essential oil**—liquids containing volatile aroma compounds—**based perfumes.** They are a safe and effective way to smell good!
- **Know your anti-bacterial soap.** Many of these soaps contain triclosan, which has been linked with endocrine disruption http://bit.ly/10EtLc5

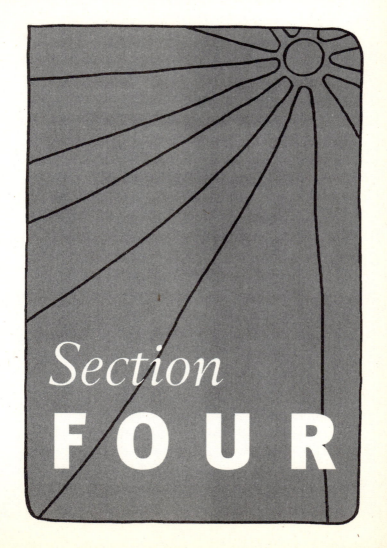

# Keeping the Body 'Tuned Up'

**(*Ikkuma* Translation: *Stoking The Fire*)**

*"Look not mournfully into the past. It comes not back again. Wisely improve the present. It is thine. Go forth to meet the shadowy future, without fear."*
—Henry Wadsworth Longfellow,
19th century American poet

The foundation of good health involves proper nutrition, exercise, the elimination of toxins, a proper nights sleep, stress management and don't forget a positive attitude. All these aspects of your daily life help create a favourable environment for you to thrive. I've already touched on the greater importance of environment, compared to your genetics, as a very important determining factor in preventing disease and maintaining overall health.

To take this one step further, the environment that you create in the body can actually influence genetic expression. So, take control of your physical well-being—helping to create the proper environment in the body—before your body takes control of you.

**SECTION FOUR:** KEEPING THE BODY 'TUNED UP' 255

Now that we've established that it is 'you' that controls your fate, what are your goals when it comes to your health? What do you want to achieve? Once you understand your goals, you need to be honest with yourself, and ask what you're prepared to do? Set your priorities and begin making a plan. And to be frank, I don't care what your goals are—be it vanity or genuine health—because living a healthy life will help you achieve all your goals.

Don't find yourself in the excuse trap where you rationalize inaction. Some will blame it on not having time because of the kids, job, other priorities, and so on, but you truly need to make health and self-care a priority. You may not feel the effects of neglect immediately, but you will down the road. You know this. If you want to take control, this next section is critical and will change your life forever. Guaranteed!

Remember that health and well-being is a life long journey. Start implementing changes that you will be able to sustain… and take it one step at a time. If you are just starting out, be realistic. The key is to make a change today.

In this final section, as we explore stress, sleep, and fitness, I will attempt to define the importance of each concept, followed by improvement advice. It is a slight change of gears, in that, we are now addressing how we treat our bodies. It will take a little more work on your part.

## Stress... The Silent Killer

> *"He who is of calm and happy nature will hardly feel the pressure of age, but to him who is of an opposite disposition, youth and age are equally a burden."*
> —PLATO, GREEK PHILOSOPHER

Stress gets a lot of press these days, and rightfully so. There is a constant barrage of warnings that stress can eventually kill you, thus encouraging you to avoid it at all costs. Despite this, the average person does not understand how stress manifests itself inside their body. For many of us, since we will only feel the serious effects of stress, five, ten, fifteen years down the road, we tend to ignore it. We rationalize our situation and convince ourselves that we don't need to change, that it's not a problem.

You need to educate yourself and start understanding what happens in your body. You need to think twice about allowing stress to adversely affect your health. Will it take a heart attack to realize that stress kills you? For many it does. Have you had a heart attack? Have you spoken to someone who has had a heart attack? Have you seen the aftermath of open-heart surgery? It's a little worse than taking 5 minutes here and there to be present and calm. And that job you pine over. If it's killing you then it might be time to take a look around at the things you love and truly assess your priorities—again, this isn't my call. Often times the effects of stress are not perceivable until it's too late; and yes, it can kill if you let it get out of control.

### i. Physiological response

*"It is the mind that makes the body."*
—SOJOURNER TRUTH, 19TH CENTURY AMERICAN ORATOR

There are many different sources of stress and responses to stress. Unfortunately, discussing the specific physiological response of stress is never black and white. There are infinite degrees of stress, thus infinite responses by your body. The sources and nature of stress have evolved over time, much like human society has, but our body's physiological response has remained fairly consistent.

For our ancestors, stress may have come from being chased by a bear. Their body's natural defenses would kick in, prompting that well known rush of adrenaline along with a rush of cortisol—the 'fight or flight' hormone. Their body's priorities would then switch from daily life—repair and digestion—to survival. Their heart rate would take off, blood sugar would spike, and senses would heighten. Essentially stress is our response to a perceived threat, which helped keep our ancestors alive. This response is then meant to be followed by the 'rest and digest', or parasympathetic, phase.

Today a bear is most likely not chasing you, but maybe you can't pay the bills, or maybe work stresses don't let up. Though there may not necessarily be life-threatening stresses, constant modern day stressors prevent many people from transitioning back into the parasympathetic phase, forcing their bodies to exist in the sympathetic condition of fight or flight.

A chronic sympathetic state leads to adrenal exhaustion, lowered immunity, high blood pressure, insulin resistance and excessive cortisol. Although necessary for survival, in excess, cortisol breaks down muscle (catabolism), increases blood pressure, and releases glucose and fatty acids from the liver. It also blunts insulin sensitivity and adds to that dangerous visceral fat around your abdomen. So, controlling your stress will help you lose that belly.

Speaking of belly, your gut is one of the main victims in this chronic state of stress. Few realize it but gut health and stress will be forever linked. Our gut has the second highest concentration of neurons, with the brain having the lions share. The gut therefore is essentially our second brain. Those butterflies in your stomach, or that 'gut feeling' are all examples of how your gut, and emotions play hand in hand. It is no surprise that chronic stress has a detrimental effect on our gut health through:

- Severely decreasing enzyme production—enzymes are essentially catalysts for metabolic reactions, like digestion
- Reducing absorption of key vitamins and minerals
- Short changing gut flora population
- Delivering up to four times less blood flow to your digestive tract, reducing metabolism

### ii. Stress Management

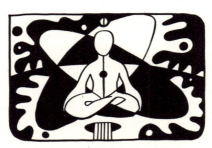

"Meditation"—"Sit in the stillness of your center and let your grounded energy radiate peace."—S. LeBlanc

*"Laughter is the most healthful exertion."*
   —Christoph Wilhelm Hufeland,
      18th Century German physician and writer

*"Never continue in a job you don't enjoy. If you're happy in what you're doing, you'll like yourself, you'll have inner peace. And if you have that, along with physical health, you will have had more success than you could possibly have imagined."*
   —Johnny Carson, American comedian

It is not a secret that diet and exercise are key for maintaining optimal health. Let's review how both of these can do wonders for stress reduction.

Diet is the foundation for all health. So, it is no surprise that stress, being so linked to maintaining optimal health, is directly affected by diet. The angle I will take regarding stress and diet's interdependency is not what you may think. Yes, substances like caffeine may induce anxiety and stress due to the adrenaline rush brought on, but the biggest concern lies in the stress the body is put under by certain foods. Refined carbohydrates, such as white bread, sugar, high fructose corn syrup, and processed foods high in salt, are potentially responsible for putting your body under undue stress through promoting chronic inflammation. Explained earlier, chronic inflammation is an immune response brought on by the body to address and heal the damage that has been created from a poor diet. Eliminate the culprits and reduce inflammation.

Besides diet, exercise can be a guaranteed avenue for reducing stress. Apart from the simple act of (hopefully) taking your mind off your sources of anxiety, exercise prompts very positive, stress reducing physiological responses within the body. Exercise produces several 'feel good' hormones, such as norepinephrine, serotonin and dopamine, which can help tame your feelings of stress and anxiety. Listening to music while exercising is also a great idea, as it can help improve your workout and your mood.

I'd now like to give you a quick exercise and a few tips on how you can leverage the mind to reduce stress. Some would call it meditation, but it can be as simple as taking the time to properly breathe. We take oxygen for granted but it can be immensely therapeutic. This exercise only takes a few minutes and can do wonders for relieving stress in the body. It will lower your blood pressure and heart rate, and inevitably, your stress level:

- Breathe in through your nose for a 5-8 count
- Hold for 1 second
- Exhale through your mouth for a 5 count
- During the entire exercise focus on all body sys-

tems involved in breathing… nostrils, diaphragm, stomach and lungs
- Repeat this 10–15 times

As mentioned, we are in a constant battle with stress in our lives, so incorporate these key suggestions to maintain a more peaceful routine:

- Be present and aware
- Be compassionate and kind to others—favor respect, dignity and tolerance
- Add sweetness to life, decrease what feels sour or bitter
- Indulge in nature—spend time in nature and appreciate its beauty
- Be calm within yourself—don't add to the agitation that surrounds us
- Be of service—not only to friends and family but those in need
- Breath deeply—from the diaphragm—avoid shallow chest breathing
- Meditate daily—I suggest a minimum of 15 minutes every morning
- Be grateful—keep a gratitude journal and update it daily

I can't stress enough (excuse the pun) how important it is to manage this silent killer. Remember that if you don't find surefire ways to combat the stress in your life then you could be at risk for several adverse health issues.

### Ikkuma Top *Stress Management* Tweets:

- Eating healthy foods is a foundation for well-being, which includes stress management. **Processed foods are inflammatory, adding to stress.**
- Take a break for **5 minutes to just breath**. Breath in through your nose, hold, and out through your mouth. This will quickly reduce stress.
- **Meditation** is often labeled as something left for the shamans and yogis. Its incredible benefits are being noticed http://huff.to/13cqNHG

### Bonus Ikkuma *Stress Management* Tweets:

- **Laughing** can have stress busting and blood pressure reducing effects. Try to get at least 5 hearty laughs daily.
- **Smiling** isn't just a sign that someone is happy. The act of smiling can help with recovery after stressful events http://bit.ly/10CKHuO

- **Outdoor exercise** has been shown to directly improve well-being, with the greatest effect in areas around water http://bbc.in/ZTnvbU

## Sleep...The Body's Time to Heal

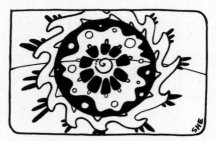

"Cycles"—"Circadian rhythms work to keep our bodies in sync with our inner workings and our outer environment."—S. LeBlanc

*"Take a rest; a field that has rested gives a bountiful crop."*
—Ovid, ancient Roman poet

There's one in every bunch who claims that they don't need more than a few hours of sleep. So what they're telling me is that after millions of years of evolution, they are the genetic anomaly that doesn't need sleep. Maybe they're the disruptive evolutionary shift that will be the new normal. I think not. Bottom line is that everyone needs ample sleep. In this section I'll illustrate you how you can get the best sleep possible.

What is sleep? This may at first seem like an idiotic question, but I am not patronizing you; there is much information regarding sleep that many are unaware of.

Adding a little context to frame things up, let's understand the anatomy of our critical sleep cycle, or circadian cycle, starting from when you wake up. In the morning, our blood pressure and temperature increase to stage your body for the day to come. By mid-morning you become fully alert and your metabolism is really ramping up, while sunlight keeps us awake and alert during the day. Your metabolism typically peaks sometime around mid-afternoon, when you are at your physical and mental best (after that post lunch nap!). Once the evening arrives, your metabolism starts to calm, and your body temperature starts to drop—all in step with increased production of melatonin. Melatonin, often referred to as the sleep hormone, is critical for regulating sleep patterns. Once you fall asleep melatonin has peaked and your body is in a state of repair and rejuvenation. This sleep cycle is referred to as your circadian rhythm.

Without boring you with too much science, I will briefly dig in a little deeper into your circadian rhythm's signficance. Everybody has an internal clock called the Suprachaismatic Nucleus (SCN), which is hard wired to the eyes. Think of this as your conductor. When the sun goes down, this "conductor" prompts your pineal gland to produce melatonin; a process necessary to keep the body synchronized, and allow your cells work in step. When you mess with this process, through inconsistent sleeping patterns and sabotaged sleep, your body is no longer in tune. Instead of Beethoven, your body has become a bad contestant from American Idol.

For whatever the reason, the reality is that very few of us get enough sleep, while even fewer seem to understand the consequences of inadequate sleep. It is my hope that, after learning more about sleep and the significant effect it has on our overall health, more of you will start to make it a priority.

### i. Why is sleep necessary?

How many times have you heard, "I don't need more than four hours sleep"? Or maybe you've heard, "I would love to get more sleep but I just can't find the time." I have questioned countless people about how much sleep they think they need. Astoundingly many people see it as a badge of honor that they don't need much sleep. Everyone seems to think they are the exception to the rule that humans need sleep. I challenge these individuals not to set their alarms, eliminate all noise from their rooms, and track how long they sleep. I guarantee it will be more than 4–5 hours. Your body knows what it needs, so give it the opportunity to get the sleep it requires to keep everything functioning as it should.

We typically hear that between 6–8 hours of sleep per night is sufficient. Research has shown that sleeping less that 6 hours increases insulin resistance, thus increasing the risk of diabetes. Other recent studies have shown that less than 5 hours of sleep increases your risk of developing heart disease and having a stroke. The American Cancer Society published the results of a study they performed on one million adults. It showed that an inadequate amount of sleep significantly increased the risk of several cancers; the cause of which could possibly be attributed to a compromised immune system.

Proper sleep has even been attributed to reduced rates of breast cancer. In fact, some studies argue that inadequate sleep, not diet, is the main cause of breast cancer in women. That is, melatonin (which is stimulated by darkness) slows down the production of estrogen, which in excess has been linked to breast cancer. Peeling the onion a little more, there is a strong correlation between breast cancer incidence and artificial light at night. It is amazing that the simple invention—the light bulb—has had such a monumental impact on sleep cycles. As we all know, Edison's creation has been shortchanging our sleep cycles with little or no resistance.

David Suzuki effectively highlights, in the documentary *Lights Out*, the detrimental effects of artificial light at night. One great example is the relationship between shift work—disrupts the circadian rhythm—and cancer. The Nurses Health Study followed over 200,000 nurses, and found that those with at least 20 years experience increased their cancer risk by 79%. Moreover, the World Health Organization (WHO) has now lumped shift work in the same carcinogen risk category as UV rays and diesel exhaust. Other studies estimate that shift workers have double the risk of getting cardiovascular disease. Even if you aren't a shift worker, this clearly shows what can happen when sleep is compromised.

## *Ikkuma* **INFO**

**Melatonin Friendly Lights:** Research has shown that the blue spectrum in light wavelengths are responsible for melatonin suppression. That could potentially be what makes a blue sky so effective at keeping you awake. This knowledge has motivated companies to start designing lights that mimic the soft white glow from lights we're used to, without the melatonin suppressing wavelengths. This will do wonders to help improve melatonin levels right before bed.

In the end, the general rule is quite logical: you want to give your body the sleep it needs to be able to sustain energy throughout the day without stimulation. Sleep is necessary and when compromised can wreak havoc on the body. Here are a few examples how poor sleep habits can have several detrimental effects on your health:

- Significantly compromises your immune system;
- Can cause migraines;
- Impairs memory function;
- Promotes tumor growth, in that melatonin suppresses cancer cell growth
- Increases your risk of cardiovascular disease

Sleep is your body's time to repair, and gives key organs a needed break. The average person underestimates the serious consequences of ineffective sleep patterns. It is virtually impossible to be healthy in the long run if you do not manage your sleep habits. Regardless of how much you work out, or how well you eat, if you don't sleep you *are* going to encounter serious health issues down the road.

### ii. How do you optimize your sleep?

Let's break down the key ingredients to a good night's sleep and focus on a few things to avoid to improve your chances of a great night's sleep. There are two main factors to a good night's sleep: following a rhythm (circadian rhythm—as touched on earlier), and eliminating all noise—mental, environmental, and physical.

The first key to consistent sleep is to follow your circadian rhythm. As explained, in a normal day, you should wake feeling rested, and later in the day become gradually more tired. As the sun goes down, and you get less and less light, you will start to produce melatonin, ideally reaching peak fatigue right before bed. Introducing strong artificial light at night has a huge effect on your melatonin levels right before bed, as it can suppress melatonin production for up to 90 minutes after the lights are shut off.

Messing with our circadian rhythm is extremely common, as a lot of people have different sleep patterns, particularly during the weekend. I'm even guilty of this. We don't live in a bubble, so I know that there are challenges in getting regular sleep. You can catch up on sleep during the weekend, to a certain extent, but even this seemingly innocent sleep change can mess with your brain's rhythm. Try to maintain a fairly routine sleep schedule to keep your circadian rhythm in tune. To ensure your body is ready to hit the hay as planned, skip the long, extended naps throughout the day and refrain from drinking caffeinated beverages too late in the day.

Both of these, along with the aforementioned late night bright lights, can sabotage your routine.

The second key is eliminating all noise. Mental noise could be in the form of stress and anxiety; physical noise could be something as simple as a chronic pain; environmental noise can include things like the lights on an alarm clock, or having your blinds open.

Yes, the minimal light from your alarm clock can suppress melatonin, even when you are sleeping. Your room should be completely free of any light. For children who like a little light at night, the best choice would be red night lights, in that they contain a wavelength that doesn't suppress melatonin.

It's important to focus on why we aren't sleeping, and tackle the root of the issue, rather than simply address the symptom: insomnia. With that said, many people unfortunately turn to pharmaceuticals to cure their insomnia. Ironically enough, according to the FDA, many over-the-counter sleep aids have little effect on improving sleep.

Even more shocking, a National Health Institute study of prescription sleeping pills showed extremely marginal improvements (on average only minutes improvement per night) versus a placebo. We're trying to medicate our way to sleep, which is not only unhealthy, it's ineffective.

Getting a good night's sleep is not as complicated as people make it out to be. Follow these basic guidelines and reclaim what you body needs to be at optimum health.

> **Bonus Ikkuma *Sleep... The Body's Time to Heal* Tweets:**
>
> - Try to **maintain your circadian rhythm**. Constantly changing your sleep patterns confuses your body. The orchestra gets out of synch.
> - **Avoid bright lights at night.** They can suppress melatonin for up to 90 minutes after they have been shut off. Dim the lights and avoid TV.
> - **Black out your bedroom.** Even small amounts of light can disrupt your production of melatonin and serotonin, affecting sleep and mood.
> - **Eliminate noise.** If you live in a noisy neighborhood wear earplugs. This includes mental noise. Try to have a calm and peaceful environment.
> - **Avoid late night caffeine,** as it can disrupt your sleep. However, even midday caffeine can affect you. http://bit.ly/10lkggp
> - **Skip long daytime naps.** Your circadian rhythm can be shortchanged by long naps. Stick to 15–25 minute naps to get a boost.

- **Deal with chronic stress.** It affects every part of your health including sleep. Anxiety can promote adrenaline and cortisol production.
- **Steer clear of artificial sleep aids.** The sleep aid market is booming despite showing marginal improvements. http://bit.ly/YQXtuH

## Bonus Ikkuma *Sleep... The Body's Time To Heal* Tweets:

- **Reduce electro-magnetic fields** in your bedroom. EMFs can disrupt the proper functioning of your pineal gland, thus affecting melatonin.
- For late night bathroom breaks, keep the lights off or **get a red night light,** since blue light can quickly suppress melatonin.
- **Cool down your bedroom**. Your body temperature drops when you sleep. Turning down the temperature in your bedroom will mimic this change.
- **Lose the alarm clock** or try to find one that gradually wakes you up. Abruptly waking up can spike adrenaline and cortisol.
- **Get a memory foam mattress**. They transfer much less energy when you are restless in bed. This helps with a restless partner.

## Fitness... Use It or Lose It

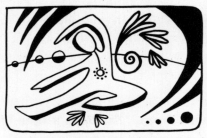

"Opening"—"Reach past where you
have been before and watch how the
world opens up to meet you."
—S. LeBlanc

*"A man too busy to take care of his health is like a
mechanic too busy to take care of his tools."*
—Spanish proverb

Let me guess, you don't have time to exercise? Don't even get me started on this one. I bet if someone slapped you in the face every 5 minutes until you found 45 minutes, 3 days per week, you would find that 2 hours and 15 minutes per week pretty darn quick. It's all about necessity. If it's a necessity you'll do it. Fitness should be a necessity. Assess your priorities and stop making excuses.

Exercise is crucial to a long, healthy and vibrant life. It's what will keep you mobile well into your later years—helping you feel younger while living longer. Besides the obvious benefits of keeping a healthy body weight, exercise reduces the risk of diseases like cancer, diabetes, osteoporosis and cardiovascular disease. It also helps to reduce depression through promoting dopamine and serotonin production, while at the same time bolstering your energy and improving cognitive function (Nordqvist J., "Lifelong Exercise Significantly Improves Cognitive Functioning In Later Life", March 2013, *Medical News Today*,). With that brief, but impressive resume, how can you not make time for exercise? Let's prime you up with basic knowledge on where to start. The rest is up to you.

Before we start, you need to understand your specific goals or basic motivation—any one of which will ultimately lead you to a healthier and more fit you. Maybe you want a beach body, or maybe just losing fat is what drives you; either way, the tips and guidelines you will pick up from this section will get you there.

You can simply modulate your intensity to achieve specific desired results. It is not unlike your diet in that there are specific therapies for specific dietary goals, yet no matter what healthy eating habits you choose, you will be promoting an environment in your body where disease cannot thrive. The same goes for fitness. Incorporate adequate amounts of aerobic and resistance training (anaerobic) into your regimen and you will develop a body that looks great, helps your sports performance, keeps you energized, and helps combat disease.

> ## *Ikkuma* **INFO**
>
> **Kids & Fitness:** It is widely believed that children should not engage in resistance training of any kind. This is a fallacy. We already know that it is very important that children exercise. One of the ways they can get this exercise is through resistance training. Obviously supervision and a reasonable workout program are important, but there is no reason why kids cannot greatly benefit from a resistance training regimen from a qualified trainer.
>
> I'm not talking about throwing them in a weight room to lift heavy weights. I'm talking about more benign methods such as using their own body weight and equipment such as resistance bands (basically elastic bands designed for exercise) or stability balls. It is more important than ever to encourage kids and adolescents to step up to the plate and get active. As is the case for adults, kids can reap benefits ranging from increased bone density and maintaining healthy body fat percentages, to improved cognitive function, reduced chance of injury, and improved performance in sports. The world has changed. Childrens' diets have become riddled with fat-producing high fructose corn syrup, and outdoor activities have been replaced with game

consoles and computers; causing the rate of childhood obesity to skyrocket. Get them active! Get them training! Their bodies will thank you for it.

## General Muscle Types

Your muscles are composed of two main muscle fiber groups: slow-twitch and fast-twitch. Slow-twitch (type I) muscle fibers are typically employed under relatively light activity. They have a high level of endurance but generate little force when compared to their fast-twitch siblings. As such it takes a very different training protocol to illicit growth. People who focus on endurance sports, such as rowers and marathon runners, would typically rely more on their type I fibers.

The second major group of muscle fibers, your fast-twitch (type II) muscle fibers, are recruited when you do explosive movements or are lifting heavy loads. Fast twitch muscles are further distinguished as type IIa or type IIb. Type IIa, which can take on the characteristics of fast and slow twitch fibres, have relatively more endurance, while type IIb can generate more force. The more you stimulate fast-twitch fibers, the faster your muscles will grow. Slow-twitch muscles do not have the same scale of growth. This distinction isn't only important for a 'beach body'. The more lean muscle you are able to build, the more calories you burn, in effect creating a fat burning factory.

Fast-twitch muscles also contain fibers that are efficient at storing glycogen. Although this is dependant on your diet, these fibers will allow for increased glucose absorption the more they grow. This in turn will help contribute to maintaining healthy insulin sensitivity and levels. When engaged these growth stimulating fibers also prompt the body to produce human growth hormones, which has been said to have anti-aging effects.

The key to activating both your slow and fast-twitch muscles is to work out at high intensity (speed, load, instability and tension), with a good combination of aerobic and resistance training (anaerobic). Initially your slow twitch muscles (have more endurance and recover rapidly) are recruited through aerobic activity, followed by the fast twitch muscles (the power center—promote growth) through efficient resistance training or any activity that requires quick and responsive movements (such as jumping).

## Aerobics vs. Resistance Training (Anaerobic)

I have been working out for over 20 years. While I have seen minor fluctuations in my weight and fat percentage,

I have generally been very lean for a male. I do this without doing virtually any conventional aerobic activity.

Don't get me wrong, I have nothing against aerobic activity. Obviously doing anything more strenuous than sitting on a couch will burn incremental calories and help you lose fat. However, bulding lean muscle mass through resistance training is key, as the more lean muscle mass you have the more calories you will burn naturally throughout the day (basal metabolism).

Even if you work out, approximately 70–85% of your calories burned in a day are during the time you aren't training (Mayo Clinic Staff, *Metabolism and weight loss: How you burn calories*, October 2011). It is estimated that, due to an increased basal (base) metabolic level, every added pound of muscle you put on burns between 50–100 more calories per day. This means that adding just 5–10 pounds of muscle will help you burn between 250–1000 extra calories per day, without you having to do anything different. The calorie burning does not end there. After a strenuous, high intensity workout, it is estimated that your metabolism is on overdrive for 36–48 hours; busy repairing and transforming your body to deal with its new demands.

If you want to thrive, if you want to maintain healthy bones and tissue, if you want to have that vibrant body that looks great, you should strongly consider incorporating some form of high intensity training into your regimen. Let's now dig a little deeper into how to effectively introduce both aerobic and resistance training into your lifestyle.

## Aerobics

On a purely esthetic level, simply doing moderate cardiovascular exercise will not sculpt the body. Aerobic exercise primarily recruits your slow-twitch fibers. As we have learned, fast-twitch muscle fibers ignite the greatest overall muscle growth. So, if a better physique, improving heart health, and reducing body fat, is the end goal—regardless of your gender—the right type of high-intensity aerobic training is crucial.

When it comes to exercise, we are all starting from different places, so it is important to be aware of your limits. Walking may be a great place to begin for those who have just decided to take this journey, though it definitely should not end there; as it won't push the body enough to ellicit significant change. It is a beginning, not necessarily the solution.

Despite what we have often heard, too much of anything, including cardio, can be quite harmful to the body. While the negative effects are entirely dependant on the individual, long bouts of cardio (well in excess of an hour) can:

- eventually cause the body to produce excess cortisol that, as explained earlier, is catabolic (breaks down tissues, such as muscles, and uses it for energy) and may lead to several chronic conditions
- weaken your immune system—too much of anything can be destructive
- actually damage the heart for up to 3 months when taken to the extreme, such as running marathons without significant training—again, take baby steps (Larose Dr, "Marathons damage the hearts of less fit runners for up to three months," October 2010, *Canadian Cardiovascular Congress 2010*, Montreal)

With that said, the general consensus is that any intense training supassing an hour, be it aerobic or resistance training, can promote the production of cortisol—switching the body from an anabolic state (constructive metabolism) to a catabolic state (destructive metabolism), and significantly compromises your immune system.

### Aerobic Training Guidelines and Benefits

One effective way to get the most out of your cardio workouts is to employ interval training. Interval training is a sprint & rest, or sprint & work method of cardio training that is both aerobic (prolonged, moderate exercise) and anaerobic (short duration, high intensity). Much like the wisdom of our hunter-gatherer ancestors' diet, we can also learn a lot about how they pushed their bodies. They had bouts of intense activity with rest periods, which is what this aerobic/anaerobic workout is effectively designed to mimic.

There are many variations of this type of workout, however they typically employ a pattern of sprinting for a short period of time at high intensity, then resting (rest method) or lowering the intensity (light-work method) for a period of time, and repeating as desired (entirely dependant on the individual). The key to this protocol is the ratio of work to rest, or work to light-work. For a beginner, aiming for a 1 to 4 ratio would make sense. Meaning that for every second of intense activity, you are resting or reducing the intensity for four seconds. For instance, a 30 second sprint would be followed by a two minute rest period. Make sure you have a proper warm-up and cool down.

Remember, the body is composed of slow- and fast-twitch muscle types; so unless you employ explosive movements, extend muscle time under tension, add significant load, or incorporate high intensity interval training in your cardio, you will be relying predominantly on the slow-twitch muscle fibers. The interval is designed to challenge the body and employ all muscle fiber types.

There is no magic formula, because there are many variations on how to do intervals. As long as you aim for 10–20 minute routines you should be hitting the sweet spot of effectiveness.

Here is a high intensity interval that I swear by for efficient and effective cardio:

- Begin with a proper warm-up before getting into the intervals. There are many different ways to achieve this. Proper dynamic stretching, with potential foam rolling, and 10–15 minutes of light cardio would be a good start. When choosing cardio equipment, note that low impact cardio machines include the elliptical and stationary bike, while moderate impact cardio would employ the treadmill or running outside (depending on the surface). If you have a beach go for it! You'll not only reduce the impact on your joints, but you'll incorporate 'earthing' (see Ikkuma Info: Earthing) into the health benefits.

> ### *Ikkuma* **INFO**
>
> **Earthing:** Earthing is basically walking barefoot. As Dr. Oschman explains in *Energy Medicine: The Scientific Basis*, when you walk barefoot, free electrons from the earth are conducted into your body. These free electrons are strong antioxidants. Since we are often wearing shoes we fail to consistently reap these benefits.
>
> We already know that antioxidants are key agents in maintaining healthy free-radical levels in the body. Free-radicals are brought on by many factors, including chronic inflammation, eating, and breathing. They are necessary for the healing process, because when bacteria have penetrated your skin, or you have damaged cells, free-radicals will break them down. However, if free-radicals get out of hand and leak into healthy surrounding tissue—an occurrence typically caused by chronic inflammation—you open yourself up to DNA damage. Earthing can be an effective way to combat this inflammation. The ideal location for earthing is the beach, as seawater is a great conductor. However, walking anywhere in nature barefoot will do the trick.

- After warming up, increase the intensity of the exercise to what you can maintain for only 20–30 seconds and go hard. Once you finish the sprint phase, rest for twice as long as you sprinted (1–2 protocol), i.e. if you sprinted for 30 seconds you would rest for 60 seconds. I repeat this cycle 8–10 times in succession, but for a beginner you may choose to start with a 1–4 protocol with fewer cycles in succession, working your way up over time. It is important to ensure you base your progress on your fitness level.

- Once you have finished the intervals, initiate a proper cool down. This could include approximately 3 minutes (depends on fitness level) of low-intensity cardio or walking, followed by some static stretching or self myo-fascia (SMF) release, such as foam rolling (see Ikkuma Info: Foam Rollers).

## *Ikkuma* **INFO**

**Foam Rollers:** Foam rolling a muscle is a great way to maintain good soft tissue and muscle health. It essentially irons out all the kinks in soft tissue, such as muscle fiber. When you train a muscle hard, you tear myofibrils (individual muscle strands), resulting in muscle growth when they heal. Over time, training may result in adhesions and scar tissue in your muscles and soft tissue. Even if you don't train, and are stationary for long periods of time, you can create issues in the muscle that can be solved by foam rolling.

> There are many techniques on how to foam roll, but essentially you start with the roller on the floor, placing the muscle or soft tissue in question directly on the roller. Apply as much pressure as you can handle and roll the area back and forth about 6 inches in each direction. Foam rolling lengthens the muscle, helping break down the adhesions or knots, in turn allowing for better blood flow and quicker recovery. The best time to do this would be following a workout. A few minutes of rolling makes a world of difference. You can get foam rollers at most fitness stores. They look like oversized hollowed out rolls of paper towel with about an inch of foam over the entire outside surface.

Here are some top-line benefits to performing intervals:

- You effectively work both your aerobic and anerobic energy systems
- After the age of 30 our human growth hormone and testosterone levels begin to significantly decline, accelerating the aging process. Intervals have been shown to naturally increase the production of human growth hormone (HGH) by over 500% (Mercola Dr, "Boosts Your Hormone by 771% in Just 20 Minutes", February 2012, http://fitness.mercola.com)

- Studies show that high intensity intervals improve cardiovascular endurance more than a purely aerobic cardio session, in a much shorter time (Helgerud J, Wang E, "Aerobic high-intensity intervals improve VO2 max more than moderate training," April 2007, *Med Sci Sprots Exercise*)
- It has been shown that it takes up to 48 hours for fast-twitch muscles to fully repair. This translates into increased metabolism and fat burning over these two days

## Resistance Training (Anaerobic)

Visions of muscle bound meatheads. Is that what jumps to mind when I say resistance training? I'm hoping, due to increased education on its many benefits, that this is becoming less and less the case. But yes, there are still a ton of meatheads at the gym just waiting for an excuse to flex in the mirror. Despite this unfortunate and pathetic display of narcissism, just chalk it up as necessary collateral damage. Trust me, the workout will be worth a bit of douche-bag shrapnel.

Resistance training, better known as weight or strength training, is performing exercises against a force to increase the size and strength of your muscles. Several studies have shown that, compared to aerobic training, it is a more effective way to shed fat.

Remember, muscles need energy to function. As touched on earlier, the more lean muscle you can develop, the higher your basal (base) metabolic rate, which in turn burns more calories at rest. This energy needs to come from somewhere. It can come from the food we eat, or it can come from the energy stores in our body—the main sources being glycogen and fat. The more energy we expend the more fat we will eventually burn off.

Let's attempt to set the record straight and arm you with what you need to start your new workout regimen today!

### i. Resistance training guidelines

I'm trying to arm you with a basic understanding of working out, so I'll need to explain a few key terms before we start:

- **Repetitions, Sets, Exercises:** there are "x" number of repetitions in a set, and "x" number of sets in an exercise. So, when you see 4 sets of 12 repetitions for a specific exercise, such as bench press, that means you are doing 48 bench presses in total. There are different rest periods and organization of sets, depending on the work-out design.
- **Volume:** I will mention this a few times. Volume

simply refers to the total amount of weightlifting during a workout.

Even though all muscles have both fast and slow-twitch fibres in varying proportions it is important to understand the science behind them. As an example, muscles like the quadriceps—your large leg muscles as seen from the front—are predominantly composed of fast-twitch muscles, whereas your smaller calf muscles are composed mainly of slow-twitch.

Just remember that explosive movements, heavy weight, tension, instability and volume, stimulate the most growth, regardless of the muscle in question. It is important to be aware, though, that different muscles do respond better to certain lifting protocols. I would encourage you to research the different major muscle groups or elicit the help of a personal trainer to learn more. For our purposes, I will keep things at a general level.

## *Ikkuma* **INFO**

**Machine vs. Free Weights:** When you load a muscle—using bands, free weights, or machines—it *will* respond. It all depends on what your goal is. If you just want to look good then it doesn't really make a significant difference. You can get bigger biceps, chest, legs, and so on by using any apparatus that will load them sufficiently (70–85% of the maximum weight you can lift one time for that specific exercise is a good estimate), prompting them to grow.

But, if your goal is overall health and functional strength, then free weights and compound movements—movements involving many different joints, such as the squat—are the ways to go. Compound movements, while working your largest muscles, will also recruit muscles that help maintain the stability needed in daily life. I try to design almost all my exercises around free weights. There are other ways to recruit your stabilizer muscles, including static or dynamic moves on instable surfaces.

### ii. Anatomy of a Work-out

I think it's important to give you a breakdown of all the different aspects of a workout, from stretching to post-workout. I'm not here to give you a personalized workout, as that would be impossible to do effectively without knowing each individual. I just want you to know how you can go about creating the most efficient work-out for you. I stress efficient. I know everyone is busy. Just like eating vegetables is the biggest caloric bang for your buck, I want this overview to educate you on how to get the biggest physical bang for your work-out buck.

*Stretching and warming-up*

Stretching is a very important part of your fitness regimen. Flexibility is one important way to help prevent injuries, however being too flexible can also be dangerous. In the end, like it or not, you're kidding yourself if you think you can get away with poor flexibility.

There are two main types of stretching, namely static and dynamic:

- Static stretching involves holding the movement for an extended period, perhaps 10–30 seconds. One example could be as simple as stretching your hamstring by extending your leg, placing it on a chair, and holding with a neutral spine.
- Dynamic stretching involves movements, where the muscle is put under tension for short periods. One common dynamic stretch is to swing each leg like a pendulum. Start with small swings and make your way up to as high as you can comfortably kick for about 20–30 swings per leg.

There is a time and place for both static and dynamic stretching. On non-training days, and after workouts, I would suggest static stretching. It is believed that static stretching before a workout can actually increase the risk of injury by temporarily weakening the muscle, and decreasing performance (Foster E., "Stretching before workouts may weaken muscles, impair athletic performance: studies", April 2013, *National Post*,).

Before workouts I would incorporate a quick round of dynamic stretches and a pre-lift routine. Pre-lifting could be many different things. It involves performing light-weight functional moves. For instance, if you were preparing for an upper body workout, I would perform a quick set of push-ups, pull-ups and potentially some dips. I would then perform a single shortened and lightweight set of each exercise (preceding the specific exercise) planned for the workout.

This routine activates or wakes up your nervous system, warms up your muscles and prepares your body for the task in hand. There are many other techiques one can use to warm-up before a training session, like foam rolling and walking. Doing a proper warm-up cannot be underestimated. It is key for exciting the nervous system. A primed nervous system will be that much more effective when called upon to stimulate the muscle systems employed during your work-out.

*Workout Design*

Personally, if I incorporate cardio into my workout, I place it at the end, and I remember to keep the total workout to under an hour. After a resistance training session your glycogen reserves have been significantly depleted, potentially priming you to burn more fat during the cardio phase; though this is dependant on the intensity of your workout, and your diet. Note that at very intense levels the body can actually burn muscle if the body isn't getting the oxygen it needs. In the end, however, it depends on your personal goals. People who are less inclined to do cardio may benefit from cardio before a workout.

Before we move on to the next section I want to explain a few things. There are an infinite amount of great programs that can be drawn up for resistance training. My focus, therefore, will not be to provide you with training programs, but to equip you with key knowledge on how to best train your muscles for strength or growth, how to stage sets, and to provide you with some highly effective exercise protocols.

One term I would like to explain is eccentric—the lengthening phase of a muscle—as it pertains to a lift. It is important to understand the benefits of the eccentric movement in an exercise. It is essentially the negative phase of a lift or when the weight is approaching the ground. For example, if you were doing a bench press or squat, this would refer to the lowering phase. There are many studies showing that it is actually this specific part of the movement that prompts the most gains in a muscle. Typically, try to focus on a 2–4 tempo, meaning you take 2 seconds on the concentric (shortening phase) phase and take 3–4 seconds on the eccentric (lengthening phase) phase to really optimize your lifts. You can use this as a general rule of thumb for most training goals.

GROWTH AND STRENGTH. Muscle growth and sheer strength are obviously correlated, however there are techniques that will allow you to focus on one or the other. It is not only the size of your muscle, or strength, that factors into what you can lift; your nervous system also plays a significant role in how strong you are. So if your goal is to lift heavy weights, you need to train your body to do so. I know, this seems obvious, but there is actually a wealth of science behind how people increase their strength. In the next few paragraphs I'll attempt to give you a very simplified overview of different training protocols to achieve different results.

If you are training for *muscle mass/growth* then you should employ in the range of 8–12 repetitions per set—and perform 2–4 sets per exercise. Try to allow for 2 minutes of rest between sets. With this type of training protocol you want to push your muscle to a point where you could potentially squeeze out one more rep in each set (just before failure), to prompt a metabolic response.

You truly want to fatigue the muscle. Your body will respond and adjust to these new demands by growing.

If *strength* is your focus, then performing 3–5 repetitions—at approximately 90% of your maximum lift—per set, will be most efficient. Again, when I speak of percentages of your maximum lift, it simply means the percentage of what you could lift one time. For our purposes, in this case, you would lift a weight that you can lift 3–5 times. You don't want to perform these sets until you can't lift any more, as you don't need to completely fatigue the muscle; you are simply conditioning your body to lift this heavier weight. Typically you should perform about 3–5 sets of a given exercise, and give yourself longer breaks—your energy systems usually require about 4 minutes to effectively recover—to ensure the muscle is well rested between sets.

Logic would then suggest that something in-between would be a comfortable split to achieve growth and strength gains. This is a simplification, however, and does not take into account the make-up of each muscle.

Typically women approach me desiring neither significant growth nor significant strength improvements. They are looking for moderate increases in growth and strength, but more importantly, they're looking for improved muscle tone. In order to improve muscle tone and endurance, employing higher repetition sets, in the range of 15–20 per set, for 2–4 sets should achieve the desired effect.

Remember our discussion on the different fibers in a muscle—type I, type IIa, and type IIb. When you want to grow a muscle you need to activate your type II fibers, especially your type IIb fibers. The best way to do this is by lifting relatively heavy weights, increasing tension or instability, and favoring explosive movements.

> *Ikkuma* **INFO**
>
> **Isometric Exercises:** Isometric exercises involve pausing for an extended period in the middle of an exercise. For instance, holding a plank for 60 seconds would constitute an isometric exercise. Belgian researchers found that performing these types of exercises tends to have the greatest effect on reducing blood pressure (Cornelissen, V.A., et al, "Exercise Training for Blood Pressure: A Systematic Review and Meta-analysis," *Journal of the American Heart Assoc.* February 1, 2013; 2(1): e004473).

There are literally millions of different ways to develop a training program. The key is to mix it up. Hit your muscles a variety of ways, keeping them guessing to keep them changing. When forced to deal with new demands they will adjust. Logical, right?

Incorporating the advice involving strength, mass,

and a combination of the two, will produce healthy muscle tone and growth—as long as you learn the proper ways to train. I recommend asking someone qualified, or getting a trainer for a kick-start. A little investment could be the life change you need.

Some women shy away from resistance training. They falsely believe that resistance training will make them too bulky. The truth is that women typically do not have enough testosterone to add significant bulk (although 'bulk' is admittedly a very subjective term). As explained earlier, an increase in lean muscle mass will burn more fat. And don't forget, muscle itself is actually more dense than fat, so when you lose a pound of fat and trade it for a pound of muscle, you lose overall size, and become more toned in the process.

SUPERSETS. I've been training for years and swear by supersets. Again, this is dependant on fitness level and experience. Supersets typically involve performing an exercise for a muscle group, and then, with little or no rest, hitting the antagonistic muscle group. Agonistic (prime mover)/antagonistic muscle group pairs are located on opposite sides of a bone or joint. Biceps and triceps (back of the arm) is one example of a pairing. Another example would be to perform an incline bench press, followed by pull-ups. After you perform a set on the bench you would take a quick break, or no rest at all, and execute the pull-ups.

One of the great benefits related to incorporating supersets into your workout is that they enable you to get a lot of volume training performed in a relatively short time. You are essentially spending most of your rest time for one muscle group, working another, so there is absolutely no excuse why you can't have a great workout in less than 45 minutes! It also gets your heart rate humming, giving you some cardiovascular work as you go. Check out www.ikkuma.com for some great sample work-outs and demonstrations of the concepts touched on throughout the section.

### *Ikkuma* **INFO**

**Post-Exhaustion Superset**

Some superset exercises can also be designed to hit similar muscle groups. Below is a more complicated, superset training protocol that I swear by, which I feel incorporates a good mix of strength and hypertrophy (growth). Admittedly, this may be difficult to follow for a beginner. It involves performing three different exercises for a similar muscle group. Each exercise is performed in series with little to no break, and the number of reps increases with each set. It is also known as a post-exhaustion superset (going from a compound movement to a more focused exercise) superset, where the sets focus on a similar muscle group. For example:

- Incline bench press (dumbbells) — 6 reps (1 second up, 4 down)
- Flat bench press (dumbbells) — 12 reps (1 second up, 3 down)
- Incline bench flys — 25 reps (control up-control down)

FUNCTIONAL EXERCISES. I am a true believer of efficiency. Heck, I'm an engineer, how can I not. Like I said earlier, our busy schedules have put enormous pressures on our free time, so if you can get more work done in less time then why wouldn't you? Compound functional exercises (involving multiple joints) is another surefire way, besides supersets, to be more efficient with your time at the gym and achieve excellent results.

Compound functional exercises recruit multiple muscle groups in single exercises, and are a catalyst for obtaining fantastic gains. Prompting multiple muscles to fire at once will, depending on intensity, set the stage for an anabolic (muscle building) response from your body. Some excellent examples are deadlifts (activates nearly every large muscle in the body), squats (blasts your mid-section and works wonders for your lower body), pull-ups (an effective judge of your fitness progress—

works arms, back and mid-section), dips (great for chest, arms and mid-section) and squats to a shoulder press (good spilt between upper and lower body).

I would encourage you look up the proper methods for all compound functional exercises, as it will allow you to learn how to perform them properly. These exercises will shock your body, eliciting a significant metabolic response.

*Post-Workout*

It is important to fuel your muscles immediately after strenuous workouts. During the workout you break down muscle fibers (myofibrils) and hopefully have used up a lot of energy. What you put into your body following a workout is extremely important as it will aid in muscle repair and growth, and reload your energy reserves.

From my experience, and from related theories, a post-workout smoothie with high quality whey protein (or other non-dairy based protein powders, such as rice or pea proteins) and some form of carb, such as frozen berries, with a liquid base, is an amazing injection of post-workout nutrients. The exact amount of protein your body needs post-workout is impossible to ascertain. However, with experience and incorporating several different viewpoints on this, I have found that approximately 25 grams works for the average man with an average work-out, while women would only require 10–15 grams. Again there is no steadfast rule. Just get some protein and carbs in you as soon as you can to support the repair process.

The Ikkuma 'Limitless' Smoothie in *Foods To 'Live' By* section is a fantastic way to energize hard-worked muscles.

Even if you nourish your body post-workout, you will probably get some muscle soreness for a couple of days. Regardless of where it originates, the faster you can deal with it, the quicker your body will grow. I'm talking about soreness, not injury. Some falsely believe it is a build-up of lactic acid that causes the soreness, but a more accepted theory is that it's brought on by micro-tears in your muscle fibers. When these tears repair, the muscle grows. Seek out products designed to help relieve and reduce the duration of muscle soreness to speed up recovery, such as arnica, or have an Epsom salt bath.

### iii. Benefits

Although the most obvious benefits of resistance training are to add lean muscle mass and attack your fat, bone density improves as well. Bones are constantly under pressure during a workout. The strengthening of bones and tendons is a physiological response to this load, potentially helping to prevent osteoporosis. Adding lean muscle through resistance training also awakens your metabolism; accelerating it for up to 48 hours after training, helping to burn even more calories, as well as increasing your basal metabolic rate.

I can't say enough about resistance training. If you haven't moved a weight in your life, start. I promise it will change your life almost immediately. After 3 months of effective resistance training you will notice incredible changes in your body. Many of you may have been jogging for years and haven't seen the results you want. Start mixing it up and the results will come:

- You'll look better, healthier, more toned
- Energy levels will increase
- Bones and tendons will be stronger and joints will be healthier
- Insulin levels will improve, and fat will melt from your mid-section
- You'll help slow down aging through reducing cortisol levels

### Ikkuma Top *Fitness... Use It Or Lose It* Tweets:

- **Kids need to be more active, get them training.** Using resistance bands and body weight, instead of weights, can safely build strength.
- **Strength training,** not aerobics, is the key to sustained weight loss. Lean muscle, boosts your metabolism, and burns more calories at rest.
- **Embrace interval training.** Sprinting combined with proper rest periods can increase your aerobic threshold and strengthen your heart.
- Aim for work-outs of **60 minutes or less.** Beyond this your body may start producing excess cortisol, with muscle deteriorating effects.
- **Walk bare foot.** Your feet receive free electrons (antioxidants) from the earth, which may neutralize free-radicals, reducing inflammation.
- **Start rolling! Foam rollers** can maintain healthy muscle by essentially ironing out kinks, lengthening the muscle and improving blood flow.
- **Opt for free weights** instead of machines to gain lean muscle. Free weights recruit stabilizing muscles, which help prevent injury.
- **Seek out a personal trainer** for gaining knowledge on how to train. With this knowledge you should be motivated enough to kick your own butt!

- Studies have shown that **brief dynamic stretching** (approximately 30 seconds) between sets increases strength. Stretch more as you age.
- **Slow speed repetitions** on the weight lowering portion of the lift (eccentric) have been shown to prompt a greater metabolic response..
- For **maximum growth** aim for 8–12 repetitions per set and perform 2–4 sets per exercise. **You grow via load, instability or explosiveness.**
- **Increasing strength** isn't just about muscle growth. It's about conditioning your brain to lift heavy loads. **Aim for 3–5 heavy reps per set.**
- Studies have shown that **isometric moves** (holding a position) or simply pausing during a repetition **may reduce blood pressure over time.**
- If you complain about not having time to train, **incorporate super-sets into your work-out** and cut your workouts by nearly half!
- **Focus on compound (multi-joint) exercises.** They recruit several different muscle groups—an excellent way to build balanced strength.
- Workouts can break down muscle fibres. **Feed your body the quality protein and energy it needs to start rebuilding!** Try an Ikkuma 'Limitless' Smoothie!

**SECTION FOUR:** KEEPING THE BODY 'TUNED UP'

### Bonus Ikkuma *Fitness Lose It Or Lose It* Tweets:

- **Count down during sets.** Psychologically it has been found that focusing on how many reps are left is motivating.
- **Avoid foods with HFCS or sugar** before a workout. It potentially reduces the amount of fat you could have burned during your workout.
- Land on the middle of your foot directly under you for **optimal running form.** Landing with your foot ahead of you is like hitting the brakes.
- **Love your dips and pull-ups!** They develop your shoulders, chest, arms, back and core, and are a great measure of overall fitness.
- **Protect your back with good posture.** For all exercises pump out your chest like a proud lion, keep you shoulders back and stick out your butt.
- Incorporate a **high volume work-out** into your regimen to accelerate growth. Look up German volumetric training for an example.
- **Work out at least 3 times per week.** I'm sure you don't treat brushing your teeth as discretionary. Fitness shouldn't be optional either.
- **Bring the iPod!** Listening to up-tempo music has been found to increase gains, as does training with a partner. http://bit.ly/ZW8sOz

- **Avoid the scale.** As you put on lean muscle your weight may increase. Muscle is denser than fat. Stick to your program—results will follow.

## In the End It's Your Choice...

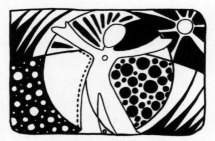

"Vitality"—"We are alive! The world celebrates with each moment of our mindfulness and gratitude for that awareness"—S. LeBlanc

*"There is nothing like returning to a place that remains unchanged to find the ways in which you yourself have altered."*
—NELSON MANDELA, FORMER SOUTH AFRICAN PRESIDENT

Before I wrap this up, I'd like you to know that I, in no way, tried to offend anybody. Yes, I have my opinions, which are sometimes strong opinions, so maybe my exuberant language is at times atomically bonded with an expletive or two. Let's chalk it up as me being a very passionate guy, who is desperate to connect with people who are ready to make a change. Ikkuma isn't a job for me. Ikkuma isn't a book. Ikkuma is my life and I'll be doing this until I'm dead. I have no aspirations of retiring. This is what I will be doing for, hopefully, the next 60 years. Yes, that will make me over 100 years old.

Most of you reading this book have the freedom to choose. At times I feel we have taken this freedom as a carte blanche to treat ourselves the way we want without any regard to its impact on the people and the world around us. Yet, we don't exist on this earth alone. We are part of communities and ecosystems. Like it or not, we are affected by decisions that our brothers and sisters make in their daily lives. If somebody decides to live a life of decadence, we are potentially paying for their health care as they prematurely succumb to disease. If somebody overconsumes without any regard to sustainability, then the environment we all rely on suffers.

I'm not here to judge. I cannot possibly understand each and every person's motivation for living the life they chose, nor should I. What I can do however, for those willing to expand their consciousness, is lift the veil of someone's individual reality and expose them to the many complex layers of interaction between all living things. Hopefully those who feel we have a responsibility for the many generations that follow ours will make positive changes in their lives, benefitting themselves, their fellow tribesman, and the nature we rely on for our existence.

Can this book make a difference? If I didn't believe it could, I wouldn't have ventured down this petrifying journey. Transitioning from a comfortable corporate life to becoming an author is hands-down the most difficult thing I have ever done. This may seem idealistic and naïve but I truly do think that Ikkuma can have an impact.

I'm approached by people all the time asking me why we need another book on health and wellness, ostensibly because they feel all the information already exists. Okay, fair enough, if you search for the information it's available. Yet, despite this wealth of information, obesity is growing at the fastest rate in history and we are being kept alive by drugs and advanced treatments.

Just to give you an example of the state of our society, here are the titles of three articles I found in today's newspapers:

- "Mystery wheat strikes fear in farmers"—alluding to mysterious, unapproved GMO wheat
- "Check your freezer: 22,737lbs of beef recalled"—notifying the public of a beef recall due to E-coli
- "U.S. doctors say obesity is a disease"—it has come to this!

This isn't an unusual day. I read this kind of stuff daily. Things aren't getting better, they're getting much worse. So, I challenge back, if indeed the secret to health exists, why the hell haven't things changed? The answer: the audience isn't getting the message in a way they can assimilate it or in a way that creates a burning desire for them to give a shit.

This is exactly why *Ikkuma: Evolution of Vitality* was written. Hopefully, through breaking down concepts to an understandable and simplified level, I have created the impetus for change, the burning platform if you will, and outlined the solutions for achieving the long-term well-being people seek.

So often in life we forget that if we're trying to make an impact then we need to connect with the audience. The key is delivering the information in the most efficient way possible, and hopefully inciting the response from the audience that you wish to achieve—ignite the flame so to speak. I hope I have achieved this with Ikkuma, I hope I have ignited your flame.

I'd like to leave you with one final thought. In the introduction of this book I elaborated on why I ventured to help people get on the road to better health. In doing so, I spoke of vitality. Vitality is a word that we often individualize, in that it means different things to different people. Yet, I would venture that most people see vitality as having the energy and health to live a long and vibrant life—essentially to feel younger and live longer! I feel that all the advice, tips and explanations in *Ikkuma: Evolution of Vitality* has given you the tools to achieve personal vitality.

Taking this one step further, I do not believe vitality stops at the individual. Along the way I hope I impressed upon you how inextricably linked we all are to the environment. Is there such thing as environmental vitality? Of course there is. I truly believe that, when we embrace the challenge to achieve personal vitality, it will create an awareness of our impact on the world around us. That is what I truly strive to do. I, along with my partner Brian, strive to create a movement. A movement whose tenets are based on becoming more aware and more responsible for ourselves, and the world we live in.

I'm not going to be moral judge of our generation's intentions, but there is no disputing that personal overconsumption and greed has gotten us to this point. I believe that if we collectively choose to make positive changes on an individual basis, then we will in turn create an environment that will allow us to live a life of abundant vitality. Follow the simple advice in this book and you will achieve an energy and health that you never thought possible. The Ikkuma way!

# Bibliography

*175 Tips to Improve Your Training & Quality of Life* (Poliquin, Poliquin, 2011)

*Ask Coach Poliquin: The Best Q&A Columns From Over Two Decades* (Poliquin, Poliquin, 2011)

*Forks Over Knives: The Plant-Based Way to Health* (Campbell and Caldwell, The Experiment Publishing, 2011)

*Foundations of Professional Personal Training* (CanFitPro, Human Kinetics, 2007)

*In Defense of Food: An Eater's Manifesto* (Pollan, Penguin, 2009)

*Liver Cleansing Handbook (Natural Health Guide)* (Lake, Alive Books, 2002)

*More Natural "Cures" Revealed* (Trudeau, Alliance Publishing Group, 2008)

*Must Have Been Something I Ate* (Kotsopoulos, Oceanside Publishing INK, 2011)

*Natural Cures They Don't Want You To Know About* (Trudeau, Alliance Publishing Group, 2004)

*Organic Manifesto: How Organic Food Can Heal Our Planet, Feed the World, and Keep Us Safe* (Rodale, Rodale Books, 2011)

*Our Toxic World—A Wake Up Call* (Rapp, Practical Allergy Res Fndtn, 2004)

*Skinny Bitch* (Freedman and Barnouin, Running Press, 2005)

*The 150 Healthiest Foods on Earth: The Surprising, Unbiased Truth about What You Should Eat and Why* (Bowden, Fair Winds Press, 2007)

*The China Study* (Campbell and Campbell II, BenBella, 2005)

*The Cure: Heal Your Body, Save Your Life* (Dr. Timothy Brantley, John Wiley & Sons, 2009)

*The End of Food* (Roberts, Houghton Mifflin, 2009)

*The Little Book of Bathroom Meditations: Spiritual Wisdom Everyday* (Heller, Fair Winds Press, 2003)

*The Metabolic Typing Diet* (Wolcott and Fahey, Harmony, 2002)

*The Most Effective Ways on Earth to Boost Your Energy* (Bowden, Fair Winds Press, 2011)

*The Omnivores Dilemma: A Natural History of Four Meals* (Pollan, Penguin, 2007)

*Wheat Belly* (Davis, Collins Canada, 2012)

*You: On A Diet: The Owner's Manual for Waist Management* (Roizen and Oz, Scribner, 2009)